Somatic Exercise for Beginners

The Complete Guide to Relieve Stress, Weight Loss, Improve Body Fitness, Flexibility and Strength

Rowe Dummett

Table of Content

Somatic Workout, also known as somatics or somatic movement, is a holistic approach to physical fitness and well-being that focuses on enhancing body awareness, improving movement patterns, and releasing muscular tension through mindful, gentle exercises. Unlike traditional workouts that often emphasize external metrics such as repetitions, sets, and intensity levels, somatic workouts prioritize internal sensations and the mind-body connection.

Principles of Somatic Workout:

1. **Body Awareness**: Somatic workouts cultivate a deep awareness of bodily sensations, movements, and posture. Participants learn to tune into their bodies' signals, gaining insight into areas of tension, discomfort, or imbalance.

2. **Mindful Movement**: Central to somatic workouts is the practice of mindful movement, where individuals engage in exercises with focused attention and intention. This mindfulness allows for greater control over movement patterns and encourages relaxation of tense muscles.

3. **Slow and Gentle Movements**: Somatic exercises are characterized by slow, deliberate movements performed with minimal effort. By slowing down movements, participants can better perceive sensations and release chronic muscular tension.

4. **Neuromuscular Re-Education**: Somatic workouts aim to re-educate the neuromuscular system, resetting habitual movement patterns that may contribute to pain, stiffness, or limited range of motion. Through mindful repetition, participants can create new, more efficient movement patterns.

5. **Emphasis on Sensation over Performance**: Unlike conventional workouts that prioritize performance and external outcomes, somatic workouts focus on the internal experience of movement. Participants are encouraged to explore sensations, such as muscle lengthening, stretching, and relaxation, without judgment or comparison.

Components of Somatic Workout:

1. **Pandiculation**: This is a key technique in somatic movement where individuals engage in a gentle contraction of muscles followed by a slow, controlled release. Pandiculation helps to reset muscle length, reduce tension, and improve proprioception.

2. **Breath Awareness**: Somatic workouts often incorporate breath awareness techniques to facilitate relaxation and enhance the mind-body connection. Conscious breathing can help individuals release tension, improve circulation, and promote relaxation during movement.

3. **Exploratory Movement**: Participants are encouraged to explore various movement patterns, ranges of motion, and body positions to increase mobility and

flexibility. This exploration allows individuals to discover areas of tension or restriction and work towards releasing them through gentle, repetitive movements.

4. **Integration of Mind and Body**: Somatic workouts emphasize the integration of mind and body, recognizing the interconnectedness of physical sensations, emotions, and thoughts. By fostering a holistic approach to movement, participants can cultivate greater self-awareness and overall well-being.

Benefits of Somatic Workout:

1. **Improved Flexibility and Mobility**: Somatic exercises can help improve flexibility and mobility by releasing muscular tension and restoring optimal movement patterns.

2. **Reduced Pain and Discomfort**: By addressing underlying muscular tension and imbalances, somatic workouts can alleviate chronic pain and discomfort, such as back pain, neck tension, and joint stiffness.

3. **Enhanced Body Awareness**: Practicing somatic movements fosters a heightened sense of body awareness, allowing individuals to better understand their physical capabilities and limitations.

4. **Stress Reduction**: Somatic workouts promote relaxation and stress reduction through mindful movement and breath awareness techniques,

helping individuals to unwind and release physical and mental tension.

5. **Improved Posture and Alignment**: By re-educating movement patterns and releasing muscular tension, somatic workouts can improve posture, alignment, and body mechanics, reducing the risk of injury and enhancing overall physical function.

6. **Enhanced Mind-Body Connection**: Somatic exercises facilitate a deeper connection between the mind and body, promoting greater self-awareness, emotional resilience, and overall well-being.

How to Practice Somatic Workout:

1. **Start Slowly**: Begin with gentle, slow movements and gradually increase intensity as your body becomes more accustomed to the practice.

2. **Focus on Sensations**: Pay close attention to the sensations in your body as you move, noticing areas of tension, tightness, or restriction.

3. **Use Breath Awareness**: Incorporate breath awareness techniques to facilitate relaxation and deepen the mind-body connection during movement.

4. **Be Mindful**: Practice mindfulness throughout your somatic workout, staying present and attentive to the sensations and movements of your body.

5. **Explore Movement Variations**: Experiment with different movement patterns, ranges of motion, and body positions to increase flexibility, mobility, and body awareness.

6. **Listen to Your Body**: Respect your body's limits and avoid pushing yourself into discomfort or pain. Modify exercises as needed to suit your individual needs and abilities.

In conclusion, somatic workout offers a holistic approach to physical fitness and well-being, emphasizing body awareness, mindful movement, and the integration of mind and body. By practicing somatic exercises regularly, individuals can improve flexibility, mobility, and posture while reducing pain, stress, and tension, ultimately enhancing overall health and vitality.

Chapter 1

Introduction to Somatic Workout

What is Somatic Workout?

Somatic workout, often referred to as somatic movement or somatics, represents a holistic approach to physical fitness and well-being that prioritizes internal awareness, mindful movement, and the integration of mind and body. At its core, somatic workout emphasizes the importance of understanding and improving the connection between one's physical sensations, movements, emotions, and thoughts.

Understanding Somatic Workout:

Somatic workout revolves around the concept of somatics, which is derived from the Greek word "soma," meaning the body as perceived from within. Unlike conventional exercise routines that focus primarily on external factors such as repetitions, sets, and intensity levels, somatic workout directs attention inward, encouraging individuals to tune into their body's internal sensations and signals.

Key Components of Somatic Workout:

1. **Body Awareness**: Somatic workout begins with cultivating a heightened sense of body awareness. This involves developing the ability to observe and interpret the various sensations, tensions, and movements present within the body.

2. **Mindful Movement**: Central to somatic workout is the practice of mindful movement. This entails performing exercises with full awareness and intention, paying close attention to the quality of movement, breath, and sensation.

3. **Slow and Gentle Movements**: Unlike fast-paced, high-intensity workouts, somatic workout emphasizes slow, deliberate movements performed with minimal effort. This deliberate slowness allows individuals to explore movement patterns and release muscular tension more effectively.

4. **Neuromuscular Re-Education**: Somatic workout aims to re-educate the neuromuscular system by rewiring habitual movement patterns. Through conscious movement and repetition, individuals can overcome muscular imbalances, improve coordination, and enhance proprioception.

5. **Sensation over Performance**: In somatic workout, the emphasis is placed on the internal experience of movement rather than external performance metrics. Participants are encouraged to explore sensations such as muscle lengthening, stretching, and relaxation without judgment or comparison.

Benefits of Somatic Workout:

- **Improved Body Awareness**: Somatic workout enhances body awareness, allowing individuals to detect and address areas of tension, imbalance, or discomfort more effectively.

- **Enhanced Flexibility and Mobility**: By releasing muscular tension and improving movement patterns, somatic workout can lead to increased flexibility, mobility, and range of motion.

- **Reduced Pain and Tension**: Somatic exercises can help alleviate chronic pain, stiffness, and tension by promoting relaxation and restoring optimal movement patterns.

- **Stress Reduction and Relaxation**: The mindful, gentle nature of somatic workout promotes relaxation, stress reduction, and overall well-being.

- **Improved Posture and Alignment**: Through targeted exercises and neuromuscular re-education, somatic workout can improve posture, alignment, and body mechanics, reducing the risk of injury and enhancing physical function.

In summary, somatic workout offers a transformative approach to physical fitness and well-being, emphasizing internal awareness, mindful movement, and the integration of mind and body. By incorporating somatic principles into their exercise routines, individuals can cultivate a deeper connection with their bodies, improve movement quality, and enhance overall health and vitality.

Origins and Evolution of Somatic Movement

Understanding the origins and evolution of somatic movement provides valuable insight into its development as a holistic approach to physical well-being.

Early Influences:

Somatic movement draws inspiration from various ancient practices and philosophies that emphasize the mind-body connection and the importance of movement for overall health. Traditions such as yoga, Tai Chi, Qigong, and mindfulness meditation have long recognized the interconnectedness of the body and mind, laying the foundation for somatic principles.

20th Century Pioneers:

The modern concept of somatic movement began to take shape in the 20th century with the pioneering work of individuals such as Thomas Hanna, Moshe Feldenkrais, and F.M. Alexander. Each of these visionaries developed unique somatic methods aimed at improving movement efficiency, reducing muscular tension, and enhancing body awareness.

- **Thomas Hanna**: Hanna coined the term "somatics" and founded the field of Hanna Somatic Education (HSE). He developed a series of gentle movement exercises known as "pandiculation" to reset muscular tension and promote relaxation.

- **Moshe Feldenkrais**: Feldenkrais developed the Feldenkrais Method, which focuses on reprogramming movement patterns through awareness and gentle, exploratory movements. His method emphasizes the importance of sensory feedback and kinesthetic learning.

- **F.M. Alexander**: Alexander Technique, developed by F.M. Alexander, emphasizes the relationship between posture, movement, and thought. Through guided movement and hands-on manipulation, practitioners learn to release habitual tensions and improve coordination.

Integration into Modern Practices:

In recent decades, somatic movement has gained recognition and popularity within the fields of dance, physical therapy, somatic psychology, and holistic health. Dance forms such as modern dance, contact improvisation, and somatic dance incorporate somatic principles to enhance movement quality, expressiveness, and injury prevention.

Contemporary Approaches:

Today, somatic movement encompasses a diverse range of practices and approaches, including Somatic Experiencing, Body-Mind Centering, Continuum Movement, and Somatic Yoga. These approaches share a common emphasis on internal awareness, mindful movement, and the integration of body and mind.

Evolution in the Digital Age:

Advancements in technology and communication have facilitated the widespread dissemination of somatic practices through online platforms, virtual classes, and digital resources. This accessibility has enabled individuals from diverse backgrounds to explore and benefit from somatic movement regardless of geographical location or physical ability.

Conclusion:

The origins and evolution of somatic movement reflect a deep-seated human desire to understand and optimize the relationship between the body and mind. Drawing from ancient traditions, pioneering research, and contemporary innovations, somatic movement continues to evolve as a powerful tool for enhancing physical well-being, promoting self-awareness, and facilitating personal growth.

Understanding the Mind-Body Connection

The mind-body connection lies at the heart of somatic workout, shaping its philosophy and guiding its practices. This section delves into the intricacies of this connection, exploring how our thoughts, emotions, and physical sensations influence one another.

The Unity of Mind and Body:

Somatic workout operates on the fundamental principle that the mind and body are inseparable entities, constantly interacting and influencing each other. This perspective contrasts with conventional approaches that often treat the mind and body as separate entities, neglecting their interconnectedness.

Embodied Cognition:

Embodied cognition is a key concept in understanding the mind-body connection. It proposes that our thoughts and perceptions are deeply influenced by bodily experiences and sensations. In other words, our physical movements and sensations shape our cognitive processes and vice versa.

The Role of Sensation:

Sensations serve as the bridge between the mind and body in somatic workout. By tuning into bodily sensations such as tension, relaxation, warmth, and discomfort, individuals gain valuable insights into their physical and emotional states. Sensations act as signals, guiding individuals to areas of tension or imbalance that require attention and release.

Emotions and Physical Expression:

Emotions are intimately linked to physical sensations and movements. For example, feelings of stress or anxiety can manifest as muscular tension or shallow breathing, while joy and relaxation may be expressed through fluid, relaxed movements. Somatic workout provides a platform for exploring and processing emotions through embodied practices.

The Impact of Thoughts and Beliefs:

Our thoughts and beliefs exert a powerful influence on our physical experiences. Negative thought patterns and limiting beliefs can contribute to chronic tension, pain, and restricted movement patterns. Somatic workout encourages individuals to cultivate awareness of their thought patterns and beliefs, challenging those that no longer serve them and fostering more supportive mental habits.

Mindful Movement as a Path to Integration:

Mindful movement lies at the intersection of the mind-body connection in somatic workout. By engaging in movement practices with full awareness and presence, individuals deepen their understanding of the mind-body connection and cultivate greater integration between the two. Mindful movement serves as a vehicle for self-exploration, self-expression, and self-transformation.

Conclusion:

Understanding the mind-body connection is essential for engaging effectively with somatic workout. By recognizing the intimate relationship between our thoughts, emotions, and physical sensations, we can harness the power of somatic practices to cultivate greater awareness, resilience, and well-being in our lives.

Benefits of Somatic Workout

Somatic workout offers a plethora of benefits that extend beyond physical fitness, encompassing mental, emotional, and holistic well-being. This section explores the diverse array of advantages that individuals can derive from engaging in somatic practices.

1. Improved Body Awareness:

- Somatic workout fosters a heightened sense of body awareness, enabling individuals to tune into their physical sensations, movements, and postures with greater clarity and precision.

- Enhanced body awareness allows for early detection of muscular tension, imbalances, and areas of discomfort, empowering individuals to address these issues proactively.

2. Enhanced Flexibility and Mobility:

- Through gentle, mindful movements and neuromuscular re-education, somatic workout can improve flexibility, mobility, and range of motion.

- By releasing chronic muscular tension and restoring optimal movement patterns, somatic exercises facilitate greater ease and fluidity in movement.

3. Reduced Pain and Tension:

- Somatic workout offers effective relief from chronic pain, stiffness, and tension by promoting relaxation, releasing muscular holding patterns, and improving overall body alignment.

- By addressing the root causes of pain and tension, rather than merely masking symptoms, somatic practices offer long-lasting relief and prevention of future injuries.

4. Stress Reduction and Relaxation:

- The gentle, meditative nature of somatic exercises induces a state of relaxation, reducing stress levels and promoting emotional well-being.

- By cultivating mindfulness, breath awareness, and present-moment awareness, somatic workout provides individuals with valuable tools for managing stress and enhancing resilience.

5. Improved Posture and Alignment:

- Somatic workout helps individuals develop better posture, alignment, and body mechanics by re-educating movement patterns and releasing habitual tensions.

- By improving postural alignment, somatic exercises alleviate strain on the muscles and joints, reducing the risk of injuries and enhancing overall physical function.

6. Enhanced Mind-Body Connection:

- Somatic workout deepens the connection between the mind and body, fostering greater integration, coherence, and harmony.

- Through mindful movement practices, individuals develop a profound understanding of the interplay between their thoughts, emotions, physical sensations, and movements, leading to a more embodied and authentic experience of self.

7. Increased Energy and Vitality:

- Somatic workout revitalizes the body and mind, replenishing energy reserves and promoting a sense of vitality and well-being.

- By releasing stagnant energy, promoting circulation, and enhancing breath capacity, somatic exercises leave individuals feeling rejuvenated, energized, and ready to tackle the challenges of daily life.

8. Holistic Well-being:

- Somatic workout nurtures holistic well-being, addressing the interconnectedness of physical, mental, emotional, and spiritual dimensions of health.

- By promoting self-awareness, self-care, and self-compassion, somatic practices empower individuals to cultivate a more balanced, fulfilling, and meaningful life.

In conclusion, the benefits of somatic workout extend far beyond physical fitness, encompassing mental, emotional, and holistic well-being. By incorporating somatic practices into their daily routines, individuals can experience profound transformations in their relationship with their bodies, their minds, and the world around them.

Chapter 2

Principles of Somatic Movement

Body Awareness: Developing Sensory Perception

Body awareness lies at the core of somatic movement, serving as the foundation upon which all other principles are built. This section delves into the importance of developing sensory perception and cultivating a deep understanding of one's physical self.

1. The Significance of Body Awareness:

- Body awareness refers to the ability to perceive and interpret the sensations, movements, and internal states of the body.

- Developing body awareness is essential for identifying areas of tension, discomfort, or imbalance, as well as for understanding the effects of movement on the body.

2. Tuning into Sensations:

- Somatic movement encourages individuals to tune into the rich tapestry of sensations present within their bodies, ranging from subtle nuances to more pronounced feelings.

- Sensations may include feelings of tension, relaxation, warmth, coolness, heaviness, lightness, and more, each providing valuable information about the state of the body.

3. Heightened Sensory Perception:

- Through regular practice of somatic exercises, individuals can enhance their sensory perception, becoming more attuned to the intricacies of their bodily experiences.

- Heightened sensory perception allows for greater precision in movement, enabling individuals to make subtle adjustments to posture, alignment, and muscle engagement.

4. Exploring Movement Qualities:

- Body awareness extends beyond static sensations to encompass the dynamic qualities of movement, such as fluidity, rhythm, coordination, and proprioception.

- By exploring different movement qualities, individuals can expand their movement repertoire, cultivate versatility, and express themselves more authentically through movement.

5. Mindful Observation:

- Mindful observation is a key practice in developing body awareness, involving non-judgmental, present-moment awareness of one's bodily experiences.

- Through mindful observation, individuals learn to observe sensations without reacting to them, fostering a sense of curiosity, openness, and acceptance.

6. Cultivating Interoception:

- Interoception refers to the ability to perceive internal bodily sensations, such as heartbeat, respiration, digestion, and emotional arousal.

- Cultivating interoceptive awareness through somatic movement allows individuals to deepen their understanding of the mind-body connection and develop greater self-regulation skills.

7. Integrating Body Awareness into Daily Life:

- The benefits of body awareness extend beyond the practice of somatic movement, permeating all aspects of daily life.

- By integrating body awareness into activities such as walking, sitting, standing, and interacting with others, individuals can foster a deeper sense of presence, connection, and embodiment.

In conclusion, developing body awareness is a foundational principle of somatic movement, enabling individuals to cultivate a deeper understanding of their physical selves and the interconnectedness of mind and body. By honing their sensory perception and mindful observation skills, individuals can enhance their movement practices, promote self-healing, and unlock new dimensions of embodied experience.

Mindful Movement: Cultivating Present Moment Awareness

Mindful movement serves as a cornerstone of somatic practice, emphasizing the importance of being fully present and attentive to one's bodily experiences. This section explores the principles and techniques involved in cultivating present moment awareness through movement.

1. Understanding Mindful Movement:

- Mindful movement involves performing physical exercises with full awareness and intention, focusing attention on the present moment and the sensations arising in the body.

- Unlike automatic or distracted movement, mindful movement requires conscious engagement of the senses, fostering a deeper connection with the body and the surrounding environment.

2. The Role of Attention:

- Attention is a fundamental aspect of mindful movement, directing awareness to the sensations, movements, and breath associated with each movement.

- By directing attention to the present moment, individuals cultivate greater clarity, concentration, and receptivity to their bodily experiences.

3. Cultivating Non-Judgmental Awareness:

- Mindful movement encourages individuals to adopt a non-judgmental attitude towards their experiences, accepting sensations, thoughts, and emotions as they arise without labelling them as good or bad.

- Non-judgmental awareness allows individuals to explore their movement practices with a sense of curiosity, openness, and acceptance, free from self-criticism or expectation.

4. Incorporating Breath Awareness:

- Breath awareness is often integrated into mindful movement practices, serving as a anchor for attention and a gateway to deeper states of relaxation and presence.

- By synchronizing movement with breath, individuals can enhance the flow, rhythm, and coordination of their movements, promoting a sense of ease and fluidity.

5. Engaging with Sensory Feedback:

- Mindful movement involves attuning to the sensory feedback generated by each movement, including sensations of tension, stretching, warmth, and relaxation.

- By actively engaging with sensory feedback, individuals refine their movement quality, make adjustments to posture and alignment, and develop greater kinaesthetic awareness.

6. Practicing Patience and Persistence:

- Cultivating present moment awareness through mindful movement requires patience and persistence, as the mind may wander or become distracted by external stimuli.

- By gently redirecting attention back to the present moment whenever it wanders, individuals strengthen their capacity for sustained focus and presence over time.

7. Extending Mindful Movement into Daily Life:

- The benefits of mindful movement extend beyond the practice session, permeating all aspects of daily life.

- By bringing the same qualities of attention, awareness, and intention to everyday activities such as walking, eating, and interacting with others, individuals can cultivate a more mindful and embodied way of living.

In conclusion, mindful movement is a foundational principle of somatic practice, enabling individuals to cultivate present moment awareness, deepen their connection with the body, and enhance their overall well-being. By engaging with movement practices in a mindful and intentional manner, individuals can unlock new dimensions of embodied experience, self-discovery, and personal growth.

Slow and Gentle Movements: The Power of Slowing Down

Slow and gentle movements are fundamental components of somatic practice, offering a profound means of enhancing body awareness, releasing tension, and fostering relaxation. This section explores the principles and benefits of slowing down movement in somatic practice.

1. Understanding the Importance of Slow Movement:

- In somatic movement, the pace of movement is deliberately slowed down to facilitate deeper sensory perception, mindful engagement, and relaxation.

- Slowing down allows individuals to tune into subtle nuances of sensation, movement quality, and breath, fostering a more profound connection with the body and the present moment.

2. Embracing Gentle Effort:

- Slow movement does not imply lack of effort, but rather an emphasis on gentle, intentional engagement of the muscles and joints.

- By maintaining a balance between effort and ease, individuals can explore their movement potential without straining or forcing the body beyond its limits.

3. Allowing Time for Sensory Exploration:

- Slowing down movement provides ample time for sensory exploration, allowing individuals to fully experience and appreciate the sensations arising in the body.

- By lingering in each movement and observing the subtleties of sensation, individuals deepen their body awareness and refine their movement quality.

4. Facilitating Relaxation and Release:

- Slow and gentle movements create a conducive environment for relaxation and release of muscular tension.

- By moving with care and mindfulness, individuals can identify areas of tension and tightness, allowing them to gradually release and soften these holding patterns.

5. Enhancing Mind-Body Connection:

- Slowing down movement enhances the mind-body connection, fostering a deeper sense of integration and coherence.

- By synchronizing movement with breath and sensory awareness, individuals cultivate a profound sense of presence and embodied experience.

6. Promoting Mindful Engagement:

- Slow movement encourages mindful engagement with each moment of the movement, promoting sustained attention and concentration.

- By focusing on the quality of movement rather than the quantity, individuals cultivate a sense of mindfulness and intentionality in their practice.

7. Embracing the Journey, Not Just the Destination:

- In somatic movement, the emphasis is placed on the process of movement rather than the end result.

- By embracing the journey and allowing space for exploration and discovery, individuals can tap into their innate wisdom and intuition, fostering self-discovery and personal growth.

In conclusion, slow and gentle movements are essential principles of somatic practice, offering a gateway to enhanced body awareness, relaxation, and mindfulness. By embracing the power of slowing down, individuals can deepen their connection with the body, cultivate greater presence, and experience profound transformations in their physical, mental, and emotional well-being.

Neuromuscular Re-Education: Rewiring Movement Patterns

Neuromuscular re-education lies at the heart of somatic movement, offering a pathway to transform ingrained movement habits, release chronic tension, and enhance overall movement efficiency. This section delves into the principles and techniques involved in rewiring movement patterns through somatic practice.

1. Understanding Neuromuscular Re-Education:

- Neuromuscular re-education is the process of reprogramming the neuromuscular system to optimize movement patterns, coordination, and proprioception.

- Through somatic movement, individuals can identify and address inefficient or dysfunctional movement patterns, promoting greater ease, efficiency, and freedom in movement.

2. The Role of Sensory Feedback:

- Sensory feedback plays a crucial role in neuromuscular re-education, providing information to the brain about the quality and efficiency of movement.

- By tuning into sensory feedback, individuals can refine their movement patterns, making subtle adjustments to posture, alignment, and muscle activation.

3. Pandiculation: Resetting Muscular Length:

- Pandiculation is a key technique in somatic movement for resetting muscular length and tension.

- By engaging a muscle contraction followed by a slow, controlled release, individuals can reset the resting length of muscles, release chronic tension, and improve proprioception.

4. Exploring Movement Variations:

- Neuromuscular re-education involves exploring a variety of movement variations to expand movement repertoire, challenge habitual patterns, and promote adaptability.

- By exploring different movement qualities, individuals can develop greater flexibility, coordination, and resilience in movement.

5. Mindful Repetition and Refinement:

- Neuromuscular re-education relies on mindful repetition and refinement of movement patterns to promote neuroplasticity and facilitate lasting change.

- By repeatedly engaging in specific movements with focused attention and intention, individuals can reinforce new neural pathways and overwrite old, dysfunctional patterns.

6. Integrating Functional Movement Patterns:

- Neuromuscular re-education aims to integrate functional movement patterns into daily activities, enhancing movement efficiency and reducing the risk of injury.

- By incorporating somatic principles into activities such as walking, lifting, and reaching, individuals can move with greater ease, grace, and confidence in everyday life.

7. Patience and Persistence:

- Rewiring movement patterns through somatic practice requires patience and persistence, as old habits may be deeply ingrained and resistant to change.

- By approaching the process with curiosity, openness, and perseverance, individuals can gradually transform their movement habits and experience profound improvements in movement quality.

In conclusion, neuromuscular re-education is a fundamental principle of somatic movement, offering a systematic approach to rewiring movement patterns, enhancing body awareness, and promoting optimal movement efficiency. By engaging in mindful exploration, repetition, and refinement of movement patterns, individuals can unlock new possibilities for movement, vitality, and well-being.

Sensation over Performance: Shifting the Focus Inward

In somatic movement, the emphasis is placed on cultivating a deep awareness of internal sensations rather than striving for external performance metrics. This section explores the principle of prioritizing sensation over performance and its transformative impact on somatic practice.

1. Redefining Success:

- In somatic movement, success is not defined by external measures such as speed, intensity, or achievement of specific poses or exercises.

- Instead, success is measured by the quality of internal sensations experienced during movement and the degree of awareness cultivated throughout the practice.

2. Tuning into Internal Sensations:

- Somatic movement encourages individuals to tune into the rich tapestry of internal sensations present within their bodies, including feelings of tension, relaxation, stretching, warmth, and vibration.

- By prioritizing internal sensations, individuals deepen their body awareness and gain valuable insights into the state of their physical and emotional well-being.

3. Mindful Observation without Judgment:

- The practice of sensation over performance involves observing internal sensations without judgment or evaluation.

- By adopting a non-judgmental attitude towards sensations, individuals create a safe and supportive environment for exploring movement, free from self-criticism or comparison.

4. Cultivating Curiosity and Exploration:

- Sensation-focused movement encourages individuals to approach their practice with a sense of curiosity, openness, and exploration.

- By allowing space for curiosity, individuals can discover new movement possibilities, release habitual tensions, and deepen their understanding of the body-mind connection.

5. Honoring Individual Differences:

- Sensation-focused movement recognizes that each individual's experience of sensation is unique and subjective.

- Rather than imposing external standards or expectations, somatic movement honors the diversity of sensory experiences and encourages individuals to listen to their own bodies and honor their unique needs and boundaries.

6. Embracing the Process:

- The process of sensation-focused movement is valued as much as, if not more than, the end result.

- By embracing the process and allowing space for exploration and discovery, individuals cultivate a sense of presence, mindfulness, and self-compassion in their practice.

7. Integrating Sensation into Daily Life:

- The principles of sensation-focused movement extend beyond the practice session, permeating all aspects of daily life.

- By bringing the same qualities of awareness, curiosity, and non-judgmental observation to everyday activities, individuals can cultivate a deeper connection with themselves and the world around them.

In conclusion, prioritizing sensation over performance is a core principle of somatic movement, offering a pathway to deepening body awareness, fostering self-compassion, and promoting holistic well-being. By shifting the focus inward and tuning into internal sensations, individuals can unlock new dimensions of embodied experience, self-discovery, and personal growth.

Chapter 3

Getting Started with Somatic Workout

Setting Intentions for Practice

Setting intentions for somatic practice lays the foundation for a meaningful and effective experience. This section explores the importance of setting intentions and provides guidance on how to establish clear and meaningful intentions for your somatic workout sessions.

1. Understanding Intentions:

- Intentions are the guiding principles or purposes that you set for your somatic practice. They serve as a compass, directing your focus and attention during the session.

- Intentions can range from specific goals, such as releasing tension in the shoulders, to broader aspirations, such as cultivating a sense of peace and relaxation.

2. Clarifying Your Why:

- Before beginning your somatic practice, take a moment to clarify why you are engaging in this practice. What are your reasons for wanting to explore somatic movement?

- Your why could be related to improving flexibility, reducing stress, enhancing body awareness, or simply finding moments of calm amidst a busy day.

3. Reflecting on Your Needs:

- Consider what your body and mind need in this moment. Are you feeling tense or fatigued? Are you seeking relaxation or rejuvenation?

- Reflecting on your needs allows you to tailor your practice to address specific areas of tension or discomfort and meet yourself where you are.

4. Cultivating Positive Intentions:

- Frame your intentions in a positive and affirming manner. Instead of focusing on what you want to avoid (e.g., "I don't want to feel stiff"), focus on what you want to cultivate (e.g., "I want to feel fluid and at ease").

- Cultivating positive intentions helps shift your mindset towards growth, empowerment, and self-compassion.

5. Setting Realistic Expectations:

- Be realistic about what you can achieve in each practice session. Rome wasn't built in a day, and neither are lasting changes in the body and mind.

- Set achievable goals that challenge you without overwhelming you, and celebrate small victories along the way.

6. Embracing Openness and Curiosity:

- Approach your somatic practice with an attitude of openness and curiosity. Be open to whatever arises during the practice, without attaching rigid expectations or judgments.

- Cultivating curiosity allows you to explore new sensations, movements, and insights, deepening your understanding of yourself and your body.

7. Affirming Your Commitment:

- Affirm your commitment to your somatic practice by verbalizing your intentions before you begin. You may choose to speak your intentions aloud or silently in your mind.

- Affirming your commitment helps anchor your intentions and aligns your actions with your goals for the practice session.

8. Reflecting and Adjusting:

- After completing your somatic practice, take a moment to reflect on how well your intentions were met. Did you experience the sensations and outcomes you were hoping for?

- Use this reflection as an opportunity to adjust your intentions for future practice sessions, refining and clarifying your goals as needed.

In conclusion, setting intentions for your somatic practice is a powerful way to enhance its effectiveness and relevance to your needs. By clarifying your why, reflecting on your needs, and cultivating positive intentions, you can create a meaningful and transformative somatic experience that supports your overall well-being.

Creating a Supportive Environment

Establishing a supportive environment is crucial for a fruitful somatic workout experience. This section outlines the key elements involved in creating a conducive setting for your somatic practice.

1. Physical Space Preparation:

- Choose a quiet and clutter-free space where you can move freely without distractions. Ideally, this space should be well-ventilated and have enough room for you to stretch and move in all directions.

- Consider adding elements that promote relaxation and tranquillity, such as soft lighting, calming colors, and pleasant scents like essential oils or incense.

2. Gathering Equipment and Props:

- Depending on the type of somatic workout you're engaging in, you may need specific props or equipment to support your practice.

- Common props include yoga mats, blankets, bolsters, blocks, straps, and foam rollers. Gather these items beforehand to ensure they're readily available when needed.

3. Setting the Mood:

- Create a soothing atmosphere by playing calming music or nature sounds in the background. Choose music that complements the pace and tone of your somatic practice, such as ambient instrumental tracks or gentle acoustic melodies.

- Dim the lights or use candles to create a warm and cozy ambiance, promoting relaxation and a sense of inner calm.

4. Establishing Time Boundaries:

- Set aside dedicated time for your somatic workout, free from interruptions or distractions. Communicate your boundaries to others in your household to ensure uninterrupted practice time.

- Treat your somatic practice as a sacred ritual, honouring the commitment you've made to yourself and your well-being.

5. Mindful Preparation:

- Before beginning your somatic workout, take a few moments to center yourself and transition from your daily activities to your practice.

- Practice mindfulness techniques such as deep breathing, body scanning, or gentle stretching to quiet the mind and prepare the body for movement.

6. Cultivating Presence and Intention:

- Approach your somatic practice with a sense of presence and intention, anchoring yourself in the here and now.

- Set clear intentions for your practice session, focusing on what you hope to achieve or explore during your time on the mat.

7. Embracing Self-Compassion:

- Create a nurturing and compassionate inner dialogue as you engage in your somatic practice. Be gentle with yourself and avoid self-criticism or judgment.

- Recognize that somatic movement is a journey of self-discovery and growth, and honor your body's unique needs and limitations along the way.

8. Reflecting and Integrating:

- After completing your somatic workout, take a moment to reflect on your experience. Notice any shifts or changes in your body, mind, or emotions that arose during the practice.

- Consider how you can integrate the insights and lessons from your somatic practice into your daily life, fostering greater alignment between your inner and outer experiences.

By creating a supportive environment for your somatic workout, you enhance your ability to fully immerse yourself in the practice and reap its benefits. Through mindful preparation, intentional presence, and self-compassionate engagement, you can cultivate a deeply nourishing and transformative somatic experience.

Necessary Equipment and Attire

Ensuring you have the appropriate equipment and attire is essential for a comfortable and effective somatic workout session. This section outlines the necessary items you'll need to support your practice.

1. Yoga Mat:

- A high-quality yoga mat provides a supportive surface for your somatic exercises, cushioning your joints and providing traction to prevent slipping.

- Choose a mat with adequate thickness and grip to suit your preferences and needs. Look for eco-friendly options made from sustainable materials if possible.

2. Comfortable Clothing:

- Wear loose-fitting, breathable clothing that allows for unrestricted movement during your somatic workout.

- Choose materials that wick away moisture to keep you dry and comfortable throughout your practice.

Avoid clothing with restrictive waistbands or tight seams that may dig into your skin.

3. Props and Accessories:

- Depending on the specific somatic exercises you'll be practicing, you may require additional props and accessories to support your movements.

- Common props include yoga blocks, bolsters, straps, blankets, foam rollers, and meditation cushions. These props can assist with modifying poses, providing stability, or enhancing relaxation during your practice.

4. Water Bottle:

- Stay hydrated during your somatic workout by keeping a water bottle nearby. Sip water as needed to replenish fluids and maintain optimal hydration levels throughout your practice.

- Choose a reusable water bottle made from BPA-free materials to minimize environmental impact and promote sustainability.

5. Towel:

- Keep a small towel handy to wipe away sweat and keep yourself comfortable and dry during your somatic workout.

- A microfiber towel is lightweight, absorbent, and quick-drying, making it an ideal choice for use during exercise sessions.

6. Supportive Footwear:

- If your somatic workout includes standing or walking exercises, opt for supportive footwear that offers stability and cushioning for your feet.

- Choose athletic shoes with good arch support and shock absorption to minimize strain on your feet and lower limbs during weight-bearing activities.

7. Optional Accessories:

- Depending on your preferences and specific needs, you may choose to incorporate additional accessories into your somatic practice.

- Examples of optional accessories include eye pillows, essential oils or aromatherapy diffusers, meditation cushions, and soothing music or soundscapes to enhance relaxation and promote a calming atmosphere.

8. Comfortable Environment:

- Create a comfortable and inviting environment for your somatic workout by setting up your space with care.

- Dim the lights, play soothing music, and adjust the room temperature to your liking to promote relaxation and a sense of tranquility during your practice.

By ensuring you have the necessary equipment and attire for your somatic workout, you set yourself up for a successful and enjoyable practice experience. With the right tools and supportive environment, you can fully immerse yourself in your somatic practice and reap its many benefits for your body, mind, and spirit.

Preparing Mind and Body for Practice

Preparing your mind and body before engaging in a somatic workout is essential for maximizing the effectiveness and enjoyment of your practice. This section outlines various strategies and techniques to help you mentally and physically prepare for your somatic workout session.

1. Mental Preparation:

- **Set an Intention:** Begin by setting a clear intention for your somatic practice. Consider what you hope to achieve or focus on during the session, whether it's releasing tension, improving flexibility, or cultivating mindfulness.

- **Cultivate Mindfulness:** Take a few moments to cultivate mindfulness and presence before starting your somatic workout. Engage in deep breathing, body scanning, or meditation to quiet the mind and center yourself in the present moment.

- **Let Go of Distractions:** Create a mental space free from distractions by letting go of any lingering thoughts or concerns. Acknowledge any distractions that arise and gently release them, redirecting your focus back to your practice.

2. Physical Preparation:

- **Warm-Up:** Start your somatic workout with a gentle warm-up to prepare your body for movement. Incorporate dynamic stretches, joint mobilization exercises, and gentle movements to increase blood flow, loosen muscles, and enhance mobility.

- **Hydration:** Stay hydrated by drinking water before, during, and after your somatic workout. Proper hydration supports optimal bodily function and helps prevent dehydration, fatigue, and muscle cramps.

- **Check-In with Your Body:** Take a moment to check in with your body and assess how you're feeling physically. Notice any areas of tension, discomfort, or stiffness, and adjust your practice accordingly to address these areas with care.

- **Respect Your Limits:** Listen to your body and honor its limitations during your somatic workout. Avoid pushing yourself too hard or forcing movements that feel uncomfortable or painful. Instead, work within your range of motion and gradually progress at your own pace.

3. Environmental Preparation:

- **Create a Quiet Space:** Choose a quiet and peaceful environment for your somatic practice, free from distractions and external disturbances. Close doors, turn off electronic devices, and minimize noise to create a calm and tranquil atmosphere.

- **Set the Mood:** Set the mood for your somatic workout by adjusting the lighting, playing soft music, or incorporating aromatherapy with essential oils. Create a soothing ambiance that promotes relaxation and enhances your overall experience.

- **Arrange Your Space:** Arrange your practice space with care, ensuring you have enough room to move freely and comfortably. Lay out your yoga mat or any props you'll be using, and remove any obstacles or hazards that could impede your movements.

By taking the time to prepare your mind, body, and environment before your somatic workout, you can optimize your practice experience and set the stage for a fulfilling and rewarding session. With focused intention, mindful presence, and gentle physical preparation, you can fully immerse yourself in your somatic practice and reap its many benefits for your overall well-being.

Chapter 4

Key Techniques in Somatic Workout

Pandiculation: Resetting Muscular Length

Pandiculation stands as one of the cornerstone techniques in somatic workout, offering a unique and effective method for resetting muscular length, releasing chronic tension, and enhancing proprioceptive awareness. This section explores the principles and applications of pandiculation within the context of somatic movement.

1. Understanding Pandiculation:

- **Definition:** Pandiculation is a three-step process involving contraction, voluntary release, and relaxation of a specific muscle or muscle group.

- **Purpose:** The primary aim of pandiculation is to reset the resting length of muscles, release chronic tension, and improve proprioceptive feedback within the neuromuscular system.

2. The Three Phases of Pandiculation:

- **Contract:** Begin by gently contracting the targeted muscle or muscle group, engaging it in a controlled manner without creating excessive tension.

- **Release:** After holding the contraction for a brief moment, slowly and voluntarily release the muscle, allowing it to lengthen and relax to its natural resting state.

- **Relax:** Finally, consciously relax the muscle completely, letting go of any residual tension and allowing it to return to a state of rest and equilibrium.

3. Benefits of Pandiculation:

- **Resetting Muscular Length:** Pandiculation helps reset the resting length of muscles by facilitating a gradual and controlled release of tension. This can alleviate chronic tightness, improve flexibility, and restore optimal muscle function.

- **Enhancing Proprioception:** By actively engaging in the contraction and release phases of pandiculation, individuals improve their proprioceptive awareness, deepening their understanding of their body's position and movement in space.

- **Improving Neuromuscular Coordination:** Regular practice of pandiculation enhances neuromuscular coordination and control, promoting smoother and more efficient movement patterns.

4. Application of Pandiculation in Somatic Workout:

- **Incorporating into Movement Sequences:** Pandiculation can be integrated into various somatic movement sequences to enhance their effectiveness and therapeutic benefits.

- **Targeting Specific Muscle Groups:** Pandiculation can be targeted towards specific muscles or muscle groups that are commonly affected by tension or stiffness, such as the neck, shoulders, lower back, or hips.

- **Promoting Mind-Body Connection:** Through mindful engagement with the sensations and movements involved in pandiculation, individuals cultivate a deeper mind-body connection, fostering greater awareness and presence during their somatic practice.

5. Guidelines for Practicing Pandiculation:

- **Start Gradually:** Begin with gentle pandiculation exercises and gradually increase intensity and duration as your body becomes more accustomed to the practice.

- **Listen to Your Body:** Pay close attention to the feedback from your body during pandiculation, adjusting the intensity and duration of the contractions and releases based on your comfort level and physical condition.

- **Combine with Breath Awareness:** Coordinate your breath with the contraction and release phases of pandiculation, inhaling during the contraction and exhaling during the release to enhance relaxation and promote a sense of ease.

6. Integrating Pandiculation into Daily Life:

- **Mindful Movement Practices:** Apply the principles of pandiculation to everyday movements and activities, such as walking, reaching, or sitting, to promote greater awareness and release tension throughout the day.

- **Stress Management:** Use pandiculation as a tool for stress management and relaxation, incorporating it into your self-care routine to unwind and release accumulated tension from daily stressors.

- **Postural Alignment:** Practice pandiculation to improve postural alignment and reduce the risk of musculoskeletal imbalances and injuries caused by prolonged sitting or poor posture.

In conclusion, pandiculation serves as a powerful technique in somatic workout, offering a systematic approach to resetting muscular length, releasing tension, and enhancing proprioceptive awareness. By incorporating pandiculation into your somatic practice, you can experience profound improvements in flexibility, coordination, and overall well-being, paving the way for a more balanced and embodied way of moving through life.

Breath Awareness: Harnessing the Power of Breath

Breath awareness stands as a fundamental technique in somatic workout, offering a profound means of connecting with the body, calming the mind, and enhancing overall well-being. This section delves into the principles and applications of breath awareness within the context of somatic movement.

1. Understanding Breath Awareness:

- **Definition:** Breath awareness involves consciously observing and regulating the breath during movement, meditation, or relaxation practices.

- **Purpose:** The primary aim of breath awareness is to cultivate mindfulness, enhance relaxation, and promote greater integration of mind and body.

2. The Role of Breath in Somatic Movement:

- **Anchor for Attention:** The breath serves as a anchor for attention during somatic movement, providing a focal point to guide awareness and promote presence.

- **Regulating Energy:** Conscious regulation of the breath can help balance the autonomic nervous system, calming the sympathetic (fight-or-flight) response and activating the parasympathetic (rest-and-digest) response.

- **Enhancing Body Awareness:** By tuning into the breath, individuals deepen their body awareness, noticing how movement patterns and sensations are interconnected with the rhythm and quality of the breath.

3. Basic Techniques for Breath Awareness:

- **Diaphragmatic Breathing:** Begin by practicing diaphragmatic breathing, also known as belly breathing, to engage the diaphragm fully and promote deep, relaxed breathing.

- **Lengthening the Exhalation:** Experiment with lengthening the exhalation relative to the inhalation, gradually extending the duration of the exhale to promote relaxation and release tension.

- **Coordinating Breath with Movement:** Coordinate your breath with movement during somatic exercises, inhaling to prepare for a movement and exhaling as you release or relax into the movement.

4. Benefits of Breath Awareness in Somatic Workout:

- **Stress Reduction:** Breath awareness helps reduce stress and promote relaxation by activating the body's relaxation response and calming the mind.

- **Enhanced Body-Mind Connection:** By synchronizing breath with movement, individuals deepen their body-mind connection, fostering greater integration and coherence in their somatic practice.

- **Improved Movement Efficiency:** Conscious regulation of the breath can enhance movement efficiency and coordination, promoting smoother, more fluid movement patterns.

5. Incorporating Breath Awareness into Daily Life:

- **Mindful Activities:** Apply breath awareness to everyday activities such as walking, eating, or working, using the breath as a anchor to cultivate presence and mindfulness throughout the day.

- **Stress Management:** Use breath awareness techniques as a tool for stress management and emotional regulation, practicing deep, intentional breathing during moments of stress or anxiety to promote relaxation and restore balance.

- **Self-Care Practices:** Integrate breath awareness into your self-care routine, incorporating mindful breathing exercises into meditation, yoga, or relaxation practices to nourish your body, mind, and spirit.

6. Advanced Practices for Breath Awareness:

- **Pranayama Techniques:** Explore more advanced pranayama (breath control) techniques, such as alternate nostril breathing or ujjayi breath, to deepen your breath awareness and cultivate specific states of consciousness.

- **Breath Retention:** Experiment with breath retention practices, such as breath holds or kumbhaka, to explore the effects of breath modulation on energy levels and mental clarity.

In conclusion, breath awareness serves as a powerful technique in somatic workout, offering a gateway to greater mindfulness, relaxation, and integration of mind and body. By harnessing the power of the breath, individuals can deepen their somatic practice, enhance movement efficiency, and experience profound transformations in their physical, mental, and emotional well-being.

Exploratory Movement: Moving with Curiosity and Openness

Exploratory movement embodies the essence of somatic workout, encouraging individuals to move with curiosity, creativity, and openness. This section explores the principles and applications of exploratory movement within the context of somatic practice.

1. Understanding Exploratory Movement:

- **Definition:** Exploratory movement involves engaging in movement with a sense of curiosity, experimentation, and non-judgmental exploration.

- **Purpose:** The primary aim of exploratory movement is to deepen body awareness, expand movement repertoire, and foster a sense of joy and freedom in movement.

2. Principles of Exploratory Movement:

- **Curiosity:** Approach movement with a sense of curiosity and wonder, exploring different qualities, textures, and sensations with an open mind and heart.

- **Creativity:** Allow space for creativity and self-expression in your movement practice, experimenting with novel movements, shapes, and sequences to discover new possibilities for expression and embodiment.

- **Non-Judgment:** Practice non-judgmental observation of your movement, letting go of preconceived notions of how you "should" move and embracing the unique wisdom of your body in each moment.

3. Techniques for Exploratory Movement:

- **Free Movement:** Begin by engaging in free movement, allowing your body to move spontaneously and intuitively without adhering to specific forms or sequences.

- **Imagery and Visualization:** Incorporate imagery and visualization techniques to inspire and guide your movement exploration, imagining yourself moving like water, wind, or a flowing tree.

- **Proprioceptive Feedback:** Tune into proprioceptive feedback from your body as you move, noticing sensations of stretch, tension, relaxation, and ease to inform your movement choices and refine your body awareness.

4. Benefits of Exploratory Movement in Somatic Workout:

- **Enhanced Body Awareness:** Exploratory movement deepens body awareness by encouraging individuals to listen to and honor the signals and sensations arising from within their bodies.

- **Expansion of Movement Repertoire:** By exploring a wide range of movements and qualities, individuals expand their movement repertoire, increasing flexibility, coordination, and adaptability in their physical expression.

- **Emotional Expression:** Exploratory movement provides a means of emotional expression and catharsis, allowing individuals to release pent-up emotions, express themselves authentically, and cultivate a greater sense of emotional well-being.

5. Integrating Exploratory Movement into Daily Life:

- **Mindful Activities:** Apply the principles of exploratory movement to everyday activities such as walking, stretching, or dancing, infusing these activities with a sense of curiosity, creativity, and openness.

- **Play and Recreation:** Embrace playfulness and recreation as essential components of exploratory movement, engaging in activities such as dancing, hiking, or playing sports to reconnect with the joy and spontaneity of movement.

- **Problem-Solving and Creativity:** Use exploratory movement as a tool for problem-solving and creativity, exploring different movement solutions to physical challenges or creative projects with an open and inquisitive mindset.

6. Cultivating a Mindset of Exploratory Movement:

- **Beginner's Mind:** Approach each movement with a beginner's mind, letting go of preconceptions and expectations to experience each moment with freshness and openness.

- **Embrace Mistakes:** Embrace mistakes and imperfections as valuable opportunities for learning and growth, viewing them as natural and inevitable aspects of the exploratory process.

- **Celebrate Discoveries:** Celebrate your discoveries and insights along the way, acknowledging and appreciating the unique wisdom and creativity of your body-mind in motion.

In conclusion, exploratory movement is a foundational technique in somatic workout, offering a pathway to deeper body awareness, expanded movement repertoire, and enhanced emotional expression. By embracing curiosity, creativity, and non-judgmental exploration in your movement practice, you can cultivate a greater sense of joy, freedom, and authenticity in your embodied experience.

Integration of Mind and Body: Connecting Thoughts, Emotions, and Physical Sensations

The integration of mind and body lies at the heart of somatic workout, facilitating a deep connection between thoughts, emotions, and physical sensations. This section explores the principles and techniques for integrating mind and body within the context of somatic practice.

1. Understanding Integration of Mind and Body:

- **Holistic Approach:** Integration of mind and body involves recognizing and honoring the interconnectedness of thoughts, emotions, and physical sensations within the individual's lived experience.

- **Embodied Awareness:** The practice of somatic workout cultivates embodied awareness, allowing individuals to witness and explore the interplay between their mental, emotional, and physical states.

2. Principles of Integration:

- **Mindfulness:** Mindfulness serves as a cornerstone principle for integrating mind and body, inviting individuals to observe their thoughts, emotions, and bodily sensations with non-judgmental awareness.

- **Emotional Regulation:** Integration involves skillful regulation of emotions, allowing individuals to acknowledge and process emotional experiences while maintaining a sense of equanimity and presence.

- **Somatic Experiencing:** Somatic experiencing techniques facilitate the integration of physical sensations and emotional experiences, enabling individuals to release stored tension and trauma held within the body.

3. Techniques for Integration:

- **Body Scan Meditation:** Body scan meditation involves systematically directing attention through different regions of the body, observing and acknowledging physical sensations, emotions, and thoughts as they arise.

- **Breath Awareness:** Conscious regulation of the breath serves as a bridge between the mind and body, facilitating integration by anchoring awareness in the present moment and promoting relaxation and self-regulation.

- **Expressive Movement:** Expressive movement practices encourage individuals to embody and express their thoughts, emotions, and inner experiences through movement, allowing for cathartic release and authentic self-expression.

4. Benefits of Integration in Somatic Workout:

- **Wholeness and Unity:** Integration fosters a sense of wholeness and unity within the individual, aligning thoughts, emotions, and physical sensations in harmony with each other.

- **Stress Reduction:** Integrated mind-body practices promote relaxation and stress reduction by regulating the nervous system and facilitating a state of calm and balance.

- **Enhanced Self-Awareness:** Integration deepens self-awareness by illuminating the connections between thoughts, emotions, and bodily sensations, fostering greater insight and understanding of one's inner landscape.

5. Integrating Mind and Body in Daily Life:

- **Mindful Living:** Practice mindfulness in daily life by bringing conscious awareness to everyday activities, such as eating, walking, or interacting with others, allowing for greater presence and connection with the present moment.

- **Emotional Intelligence:** Develop emotional intelligence by recognizing and accepting your emotions without judgment, allowing them to be felt and expressed authentically while maintaining self-regulation and balance.

- **Embodied Decision-Making:** Make decisions from an embodied place of wisdom and intuition, tuning into the physical sensations and emotional cues that arise in the body to guide your choices and actions.

6. Cultivating Integration in Somatic Workout:

- **Body-Mind Centering:** Engage in body-mind centering practices to deepen integration by exploring the connections between physical structures, movement patterns, and psychological states.

- **Journaling and Reflection:** Journaling and reflection provide opportunities for integration by articulating and processing thoughts, emotions, and physical sensations, fostering greater self-awareness and insight.

- **Group Practices:** Participate in group somatic practices and therapeutic modalities, such as somatic experiencing or mindfulness-based stress reduction, to cultivate a sense of shared connection and collective healing within a supportive community.

In conclusion, the integration of mind and body is a central principle in somatic workout, facilitating a holistic approach to health and well-being. By cultivating mindfulness, emotional regulation, and somatic awareness, individuals can deepen their connection with themselves and others, fostering greater wholeness, unity, and vitality in their lives.

Chapter 5

Somatic Exercises for Mobility and Flexibility

Head-to-Toe Body Scan: Releasing Tension Throughout the Body

The head-to-toe body scan is a foundational somatic exercise designed to release tension, increase body awareness, and promote relaxation throughout the entire body. This section provides a detailed exploration of the head-to-toe body scan technique and its benefits within the context of somatic workout.

1. Understanding the Head-to-Toe Body Scan:

- **Overview:** The head-to-toe body scan is a mindfulness-based practice that involves systematically directing attention through different regions of the body, observing and releasing tension, and cultivating a deep sense of relaxation.

- **Purpose:** The primary aim of the head-to-toe body scan is to increase body awareness, promote relaxation, and release accumulated tension and stress held within the body.

2. Techniques for the Head-to-Toe Body Scan:

- **Preparation:** Find a comfortable lying position on your back, such as savasana (corpse pose) in yoga, with your arms by your sides and your legs extended. Close your eyes and take a few deep breaths to center yourself and prepare for the practice.

- **Systematic Attention:** Begin at the crown of your head and systematically move your attention downward through different regions of the body, such as the forehead, eyes, cheeks, jaw, neck, shoulders, chest, arms, abdomen, pelvis, legs, and feet.

- **Observation and Release:** As you focus on each body part, observe any sensations, tensions, or areas of discomfort that arise. With each exhale, consciously release any tension or tightness you notice, allowing the muscles to soften and relax.

- **Gentle Movement:** If you encounter areas of particularly tight or tense muscles, you may gently move or stretch the body part to encourage further release and relaxation. Move mindfully and slowly, honoring your body's limits and avoiding any forceful or jerky movements.

- **Breath Awareness:** Throughout the body scan, maintain awareness of your breath, using it as a anchor to stay present and centered. Allow the breath to guide you through each body part, syncing your inhalations and exhalations with the movement of attention and release of tension.

3. Benefits of the Head-to-Toe Body Scan:

- **Increased Body Awareness:** The head-to-toe body scan deepens body awareness by bringing attention to the subtle sensations and tensions present throughout the body, fostering a greater sense of connection and presence.

- **Stress Reduction:** By systematically releasing tension and promoting relaxation, the body scan helps reduce stress levels, calm the nervous system, and induce a state of deep relaxation and tranquility.

- **Improved Sleep Quality:** Practicing the body scan before bedtime can promote better sleep quality by relaxing the body and quieting the mind, allowing for a more restful and rejuvenating sleep experience.

4. Integrating the Head-to-Toe Body Scan into Daily Life:

- **Morning Routine:** Incorporate the body scan into your morning routine as a gentle way to wake up the body and prepare for the day ahead, setting a positive tone for your day.

- **Stress Management:** Use the body scan as a tool for stress management throughout the day, taking a few moments to pause, breathe, and release tension whenever you feel overwhelmed or stressed.

- **Evening Wind-Down:** Practice the body scan as part of your evening wind-down routine to relax the body and mind before bedtime, promoting a peaceful transition into sleep.

5. Advanced Variations of the Body Scan:

- **Progressive Relaxation:** Combine the body scan with progressive relaxation techniques, systematically tensing and releasing different muscle groups throughout the body to enhance relaxation and release tension.

- **Body Sensing:** Deepen body awareness and presence by incorporating body sensing practices into the body scan, such as visualizing the internal structures of the body or imagining a wave of relaxation flowing through each body part.

In summary, the head-to-toe body scan is a powerful somatic exercise for promoting relaxation, increasing body awareness, and releasing tension throughout the body. By incorporating this practice into your somatic workout routine and daily life, you can experience profound benefits for your physical, mental, and emotional well-being.

Joint Mobilization: Enhancing Range of Motion

Joint mobilization is a vital somatic exercise aimed at improving the range of motion, flexibility, and fluidity of movement within the body. This section explores the principles, techniques, and benefits of joint mobilization exercises within the context of somatic workout.

1. Understanding Joint Mobilization:

- **Overview:** Joint mobilization involves gently moving a joint through its full range of motion to increase flexibility, reduce stiffness, and improve overall joint health.

- **Purpose:** The primary aim of joint mobilization exercises is to enhance joint function, proprioception, and mobility, thereby promoting optimal movement patterns and reducing the risk of injury.

2. Techniques for Joint Mobilization:

- **Active Range of Motion (ROM):** Perform active ROM exercises by moving the joint through its full range of motion using muscular effort without assistance from external forces.

- **Passive Range of Motion:** Utilize passive ROM exercises to move the joint through its full range of motion with the assistance of external forces, such as a therapist, partner, or resistance band.

- **Pulsing Movements:** Incorporate pulsing movements into joint mobilization exercises, gently oscillating the joint through its range of motion to encourage relaxation and release tension.

- **Dynamic Stretching:** Integrate dynamic stretching techniques, such as leg swings, arm circles, or trunk rotations, to mobilize the joints and warm up the muscles before engaging in more intense physical activity.

3. Benefits of Joint Mobilization:

- **Improved Flexibility:** Joint mobilization exercises increase flexibility by lengthening muscles, ligaments, and tendons surrounding the joint, allowing for greater range of motion and movement efficiency.

- **Enhanced Joint Health:** Regular joint mobilization helps maintain joint health by promoting synovial fluid circulation, lubricating the joint surfaces, and preventing stiffness and degeneration.

- **Injury Prevention:** By improving joint mobility and flexibility, joint mobilization exercises reduce the risk of musculoskeletal injuries caused by restricted movement patterns or compensatory mechanisms.

4. Integrating Joint Mobilization into Somatic Workout:

- **Full-Body Mobilization:** Incorporate joint mobilization exercises that target major joints throughout the body, including the neck, shoulders, spine, hips, knees, and ankles, to promote overall mobility and flexibility.

- **Mindful Movement:** Practice joint mobilization exercises mindfully, paying attention to the sensations and feedback from your body as you move each joint through its range of motion.

- **Progressive Overload:** Gradually increase the intensity and duration of joint mobilization exercises over time to progressively challenge and improve joint mobility and flexibility.

5. Precautions and Considerations:

- **Respect Range of Motion:** Honor your body's limitations and avoid forcing joints beyond their natural range of motion, which could lead to injury or joint damage.

- **Modify as Needed:** Modify joint mobilization exercises to suit your individual needs and abilities, using props, supports, or alternative techniques as necessary to ensure safety and comfort.

- **Consult a Professional:** If you have any pre-existing medical conditions or concerns about joint health, consult with a healthcare professional or qualified fitness instructor before engaging in joint mobilization exercises.

6. Advanced Applications of Joint Mobilization:

- **Myofascial Release:** Combine joint mobilization with myofascial release techniques, such as foam rolling or self-massage, to address muscular tension and adhesions that may restrict joint mobility.

- **Proprioceptive Neuromuscular Facilitation (PNF):** Integrate PNF stretching techniques into joint mobilization exercises to enhance flexibility and neuromuscular control through facilitated stretching and contraction of muscles.

In conclusion, joint mobilization is a foundational somatic exercise for improving mobility, flexibility, and joint health. By incorporating joint mobilization exercises into your somatic workout routine and practicing them mindfully and progressively, you can enhance your overall movement quality, reduce the risk of injury, and optimize your physical performance and well-being.

Spinal Waves: Promoting Spinal Flexibility and Fluidity

Spinal waves are a dynamic somatic exercise aimed at promoting spinal flexibility, mobility, and fluidity of movement. This section explores the principles, techniques, benefits, and applications of spinal waves within the context of somatic workout.

1. Understanding Spinal Waves:

- **Overview:** Spinal waves involve fluid, undulating movements of the spine, resembling the natural waves of the ocean. These movements engage the entire spinal column, from the cervical to the lumbar region, promoting flexibility and mobility throughout the spine.

- **Purpose:** The primary aim of spinal waves is to increase spinal flexibility, release tension, and improve overall movement quality by encouraging smooth, wave-like motions of the spine.

2. Techniques for Performing Spinal Waves:

- **Segmental Movement:** Initiate spinal waves by sequentially articulating each segment of the spine, starting from the cervical vertebrae and moving down to the lumbar spine.

- **Initiating from the Pelvis:** Begin the movement by tilting the pelvis forward (anterior pelvic tilt), allowing the wave-like motion to propagate smoothly up the spine.

- **Sequential Extension and Flexion:** Coordinate the extension and flexion of each spinal segment to create a wave-like motion, moving from a position of slight extension to flexion and back again in a fluid, rhythmic manner.

- **Breath Coordination:** Coordinate your breath with the movement of the spine, inhaling as you extend the spine and exhaling as you flex the spine, syncing your breath with the natural rhythm of the waves.

3. Benefits of Spinal Waves:

- **Improved Spinal Flexibility:** Spinal waves increase the flexibility of the spine by mobilizing the vertebrae, intervertebral discs, and surrounding soft tissues, reducing stiffness and promoting a greater range of motion.

- **Enhanced Body Awareness:** Practicing spinal waves deepens body awareness by encouraging individuals to tune into the sensations and movements of the spine, fostering a greater connection between mind and body.

- **Release of Tension:** The fluid, undulating movements of spinal waves help release tension and stress held within the spine, promoting relaxation and reducing muscular tightness and discomfort.

4. Integrating Spinal Waves into Somatic Workout:

- **Warm-Up Routine:** Include spinal waves as part of your warm-up routine to prepare the spine for more intense physical activity, lubricating the joints and priming the muscles for movement.

- **Standalone Practice:** Dedicate a portion of your somatic workout session to practicing spinal waves, focusing on the quality and fluidity of movement while maintaining a sense of relaxation and ease.

- **Mindful Movement:** Approach spinal waves with mindfulness and presence, paying attention to the sensations, breath, and subtle nuances of movement as you undulate the spine.

5. Precautions and Considerations:

- **Respect Individual Limitations:** Honor your body's limitations and avoid forcing the spine into positions that cause discomfort or pain. Move mindfully and gently, listening to your body's feedback and adjusting the intensity of the movement as needed.

- **Modify as Necessary:** Modify spinal wave movements to suit your individual needs and abilities, adapting the range of motion, speed, and intensity of the waves to accommodate your current level of flexibility and comfort.

- **Seek Professional Guidance:** If you have any pre-existing spinal conditions or concerns about spinal health, consult with a healthcare professional or qualified fitness instructor before engaging in spinal wave exercises.

6. Advanced Variations of Spinal Waves:

- **Multidirectional Waves:** Explore multidirectional spinal waves, incorporating lateral and diagonal movements of the spine to further challenge and mobilize different planes of motion.

- **Integration with Breathwork:** Integrate breathwork techniques, such as pranayama or diaphragmatic breathing, into spinal wave movements to deepen relaxation and enhance body-mind connection.

In conclusion, spinal waves are a dynamic somatic exercise that promotes spinal flexibility, mobility, and fluidity of movement. By incorporating spinal waves into your somatic workout routine and practicing them mindfully and progressively, you can enhance your spinal health, improve movement quality, and experience greater freedom and ease in your body.

Hip Opener Series: Improving Hip Mobility and Functionality

The hip opener series is a comprehensive set of somatic exercises aimed at enhancing hip mobility, flexibility, and functionality. This section explores the principles, techniques, benefits, and applications of the hip opener series within the context of somatic workout.

1. Understanding the Hip Opener Series:

- **Overview:** The hip opener series comprises a variety of exercises designed to target the muscles, ligaments, and connective tissues surrounding the hips, promoting greater range of motion and ease of movement in this crucial joint complex.

- **Purpose:** The primary aim of the hip opener series is to improve hip mobility, release tension, and alleviate discomfort or stiffness in the hip region, thereby enhancing overall movement quality and functionality.

2. Techniques for Performing the Hip Opener Series:

- **Dynamic Stretching:** Incorporate dynamic stretching movements to warm up the hip muscles and prepare them for deeper stretching and mobilization.

- **Static Stretching:** Hold static stretches targeting key hip muscles, such as the hip flexors, adductors, abductors, and rotators, to lengthen and release tension in these muscle groups.

- **Pulsing Movements:** Integrate pulsing movements into hip opener exercises to gently oscillate the hips through their range of motion, promoting relaxation and increasing flexibility.

- **Somatic Movement:** Engage in somatic movement explorations that involve fluid, exploratory movements of the hips, encouraging greater body awareness and proprioception.

3. Benefits of the Hip Opener Series:

- **Improved Hip Mobility:** The hip opener series enhances hip mobility by increasing flexibility and range of motion in the hip joint, allowing for smoother and more efficient movement patterns.

- **Alleviation of Discomfort:** Regular practice of hip opener exercises can help alleviate discomfort, tension, or stiffness in the hip region, reducing the risk of hip-related injuries and promoting overall musculoskeletal health.

- **Enhanced Functional Movement:** By improving hip mobility and functionality, the hip opener series enhances functional movement patterns such as walking, running, squatting, and bending, optimizing performance in daily activities and athletic endeavors.

4. Integrating the Hip Opener Series into Somatic Workout:

- **Comprehensive Warm-Up:** Begin your somatic workout session with the hip opener series to prepare the hips for more intense physical activity, increasing blood flow, lubricating the joints, and priming the muscles for movement.

- **Standalone Practice:** Dedicate a portion of your workout session to exclusively focusing on the hip opener series, allowing ample time to explore different stretches and movements and to deepen your body awareness and connection with the hips.

- **Post-Workout Cool Down:** Conclude your workout session with the hip opener series to promote relaxation, release tension, and facilitate recovery in the hip muscles and joints.

5. Precautions and Considerations:

- **Respect Individual Limitations:** Listen to your body and respect its limitations when performing hip opener exercises, avoiding any movements or stretches that cause pain or discomfort.

- **Gradual Progression:** Progress gradually in your hip opener practice, gradually increasing the intensity and duration of stretches and movements over time to avoid overstretching or straining the hip muscles and ligaments.

- **Mindful Awareness:** Cultivate mindful awareness as you perform hip opener exercises, paying attention to the sensations, breath, and subtle nuances of movement in the hip region, and adjusting your practice accordingly to ensure safety and effectiveness.

6. Advanced Variations of the Hip Opener Series:

- **Proprioceptive Challenges:** Integrate proprioceptive challenges into the hip opener series, such as standing on unstable surfaces or incorporating balance exercises, to enhance neuromuscular control and stability around the hips.

- **Functional Movement Patterns:** Incorporate functional movement patterns into the hip opener series, such as lunges, squats, or hip circles, to simulate real-life movements and promote greater integration of hip mobility into daily activities.

In conclusion, the hip opener series is a valuable component of somatic workout for improving hip mobility, flexibility, and functionality. By incorporating the hip opener series into your workout routine and practicing it mindfully and progressively, you can enhance your hip health, optimize movement quality, and experience greater freedom and ease in your body.

Chapter 6

Somatic Exercises for Pain Relief

Neck and Shoulder Release: Alleviating Tension and Discomfort

Neck and shoulder release exercises are essential somatic techniques aimed at alleviating tension, reducing discomfort, and promoting relaxation in the neck and shoulder region. This section delves into the principles, techniques, benefits, and applications of neck and shoulder release within the context of somatic practice.

1. Understanding Neck and Shoulder Release:

- **Overview:** Neck and shoulder release exercises involve gentle movements and stretches designed to target the muscles, fascia, and joints of the neck, shoulders, and upper back.

- **Purpose:** The primary aim of neck and shoulder release is to relieve tension, decrease muscular tightness, and improve range of motion in the neck and shoulder region, thereby alleviating discomfort and promoting overall musculoskeletal health.

2. Techniques for Performing Neck and Shoulder Release:

- **Self-Massage:** Use self-massage techniques, such as kneading, compression, and circular friction, to release tension and increase blood flow to the muscles of the neck and shoulders.

- **Static Stretching:** Perform static stretches targeting key muscles of the neck and shoulders, including the trapezius, levator scapulae, scalenes, and sternocleidomastoid, to lengthen and relax these muscle groups.

- **Joint Mobilization:** Incorporate gentle joint mobilization movements to improve mobility and decrease stiffness in the cervical spine and shoulder joints.

- **Breathwork:** Coordinate your breath with the movements and stretches of neck and shoulder release exercises, using deep, diaphragmatic breathing to enhance relaxation and promote a sense of calm.

3. Benefits of Neck and Shoulder Release:

- **Tension Relief:** Neck and shoulder release exercises provide immediate relief from muscular tension and tightness in the neck, shoulders, and upper back, reducing discomfort and promoting relaxation.

- **Improved Posture:** Regular practice of neck and shoulder release helps correct imbalances and asymmetries in the neck and shoulder region, promoting better alignment and posture.

- **Stress Reduction:** By targeting areas of the body where stress and tension often accumulate, neck and shoulder release exercises promote relaxation and reduce the physiological effects of stress on the body and mind.

4. Integrating Neck and Shoulder Release into Somatic Practice:

- **Daily Maintenance:** Incorporate neck and shoulder release exercises into your daily routine as part of a comprehensive self-care regimen to prevent the buildup of tension and discomfort in the neck and shoulder region.

- **Pre-Workout Warm-Up:** Perform neck and shoulder release exercises as part of your warm-up routine before engaging in more intense physical activity, preparing the muscles and joints for movement and reducing the risk of injury.

- **Post-Workout Recovery:** Use neck and shoulder release exercises as part of your post-workout cooldown to facilitate recovery, release tension, and promote relaxation in the muscles and joints of the neck and shoulders.

5. Precautions and Considerations:

- **Gentle Approach:** Approach neck and shoulder release exercises with gentleness and sensitivity, avoiding any movements or stretches that cause pain or discomfort.

- **Gradual Progression:** Progress gradually in your neck and shoulder release practice, increasing the intensity and duration of stretches and movements over time as your muscles become more relaxed and flexible.

- **Individual Variation:** Respect your body's individual needs and limitations when performing neck and shoulder release exercises, modifying the exercises as necessary to suit your comfort level and physical condition.

6. Advanced Variations of Neck and Shoulder Release:

- **Proprioceptive Challenges:** Integrate proprioceptive challenges into neck and shoulder release exercises, such as balancing on an unstable surface or performing movements with closed eyes, to enhance neuromuscular control and stability in the neck and shoulder region.

- **Therapeutic Tools:** Use therapeutic tools such as foam rollers, massage balls, or handheld massagers to enhance the effectiveness of neck and shoulder release exercises and target specific areas of tension and discomfort.

In summary, neck and shoulder release exercises are invaluable somatic techniques for alleviating tension, reducing discomfort, and promoting relaxation in the neck and shoulder region. By incorporating neck and shoulder release into your somatic practice and performing the exercises mindfully and regularly, you can experience significant improvements in neck and shoulder mobility, comfort, and overall well-being.

Lower Back Care: Relieving Chronic Back Pain

Lower back care exercises are fundamental somatic practices aimed at alleviating chronic back pain, promoting spinal health, and improving overall well-being. This section explores the principles, techniques, benefits, and applications of lower back care within the context of somatic workout.

1. Understanding Lower Back Care:

- **Overview:** Lower back care exercises focus on strengthening, mobilizing, and stabilizing the muscles, joints, and connective tissues of the lumbar spine and pelvis to alleviate chronic back pain and prevent future injuries.

- **Purpose:** The primary aim of lower back care is to address the underlying causes of chronic back pain, such as muscle imbalances, poor posture, and restricted movement patterns, by restoring optimal function and alignment to the lumbar spine and surrounding structures.

2. Techniques for Performing Lower Back Care:

- **Core Strengthening:** Engage in core strengthening exercises targeting the deep stabilizing muscles of the abdomen, pelvis, and lower back, such as pelvic tilts, abdominal bracing, and bridging exercises, to provide support and stability to the lumbar spine.

- **Spinal Mobilization:** Perform spinal mobilization exercises to increase mobility and flexibility in the lumbar spine, including gentle spinal twists, side bends, and forward folds, to release tension and improve range of motion.

- **Hip Flexor Stretching:** Stretch tight hip flexor muscles, such as the iliopsoas and rectus femoris, to alleviate tension and reduce compression on the lumbar spine, promoting better alignment and posture.

- **Pelvic Alignment:** Practice pelvic alignment exercises, such as pelvic tilts and hip hinging movements, to optimize pelvic positioning and reduce strain on the lower back during daily activities and movements.

3. Benefits of Lower Back Care:

- **Pain Relief:** Lower back care exercises provide effective relief from chronic back pain by addressing muscular imbalances, improving spinal mobility, and promoting better alignment and posture.

- **Prevention of Injury:** Regular practice of lower back care helps prevent future back injuries by strengthening the muscles that support the lumbar spine, increasing flexibility in the spine and pelvis, and promoting healthy movement patterns.

- **Improved Functional Movement:** By enhancing core strength, spinal mobility, and pelvic alignment, lower back care exercises improve functional movement patterns such as bending, lifting, and twisting, optimizing performance in daily activities and reducing the risk of injury.

4. Integrating Lower Back Care into Somatic Practice:

- **Daily Maintenance:** Incorporate lower back care exercises into your daily routine as part of a comprehensive self-care regimen to maintain spinal health and prevent the recurrence of back pain.

- **Pre-Workout Preparation:** Perform lower back care exercises as part of your pre-workout warm-up routine to prepare the muscles and joints of the lumbar spine and pelvis for physical activity, reducing the risk of strain or injury.

- **Post-Workout Recovery:** Use lower back care exercises as part of your post-workout cooldown to promote relaxation, release tension, and facilitate recovery in the muscles and joints of the lower back and pelvis.

5. Precautions and Considerations:

- **Listen to Your Body:** Pay attention to your body's signals and avoid any movements or stretches that cause pain or discomfort in the lower back or pelvis.

- **Modify as Needed:** Modify lower back care exercises to suit your individual needs and abilities, adjusting the range of motion, intensity, and duration of the exercises as necessary to ensure safety and comfort.

- **Consult a Professional:** If you have a history of chronic back pain or back injuries, consult with a healthcare professional or qualified fitness instructor before starting a lower back care program to ensure that the exercises are appropriate for your condition and goals.

6. Advanced Variations of Lower Back Care:

- **Proprioceptive Challenges:** Integrate proprioceptive challenges into lower back care exercises, such as performing movements on unstable surfaces or incorporating balance exercises, to enhance neuromuscular control and stability in the lumbar spine and pelvis.

- **Functional Movement Integration:** Incorporate functional movement patterns into lower back care exercises, such as squats, lunges, or deadlifts, to simulate real-life movements and promote greater integration of core strength and stability into daily activities.

In summary, lower back care exercises are essential somatic practices for relieving chronic back pain, promoting spinal health, and improving overall well-being. By incorporating lower back care into your somatic workout routine and practicing the exercises mindfully and regularly, you can experience significant improvements in lower back comfort, mobility, and function.

Release for Tight Hips: Easing Hip Tension and Stiffness

Somatic exercises tailored to release tight hips are pivotal for mitigating discomfort, enhancing flexibility, and fostering better mobility in the hip region. This segment navigates through the principles, methodologies, advantages, and implementations of hip release within the somatic workout framework.

1. Understanding Release for Tight Hips:

- **Overview:** Release exercises for tight hips are designed to address muscular tension and stiffness in the hip flexors, adductors, abductors, and external rotators, facilitating relaxation and increased range of motion in the hip joint.

- **Purpose:** The primary objective of hip release exercises is to alleviate discomfort, enhance flexibility, and promote freedom of movement in the hip region, contributing to overall musculoskeletal health and well-being.

2. Techniques for Performing Release for Tight Hips:

- **Self-Myofascial Release (SMR):** Employ SMR techniques using foam rollers, massage balls, or specialized tools to target trigger points and release tension in the muscles and fascia surrounding the hips.

- **Static Stretching:** Engage in static stretches that specifically target tight hip muscles, such as the hip flexors (iliopsoas), piriformis, glutes, and hamstrings, to lengthen and relax these muscle groups.

- **Dynamic Mobilization:** Incorporate dynamic mobilization movements, such as hip circles, leg swings, and hip hinges, to gently mobilize the hip joint and surrounding tissues, promoting increased blood flow and flexibility.

- **Breath Awareness:** Practice deep, diaphragmatic breathing to enhance relaxation and facilitate the release of tension in the hip muscles and connective tissues during stretching and mobilization exercises.

3. Benefits of Release for Tight Hips:

- **Increased Flexibility:** Release exercises for tight hips improve flexibility by releasing muscular tension and increasing the elasticity of the hip muscles and connective tissues, allowing for a greater range of motion in hip movements.

- **Pain Reduction:** By alleviating tightness and stiffness in the hip region, release exercises help reduce pain and discomfort associated with conditions such as hip impingement, IT band syndrome, and piriformis syndrome.

- **Enhanced Mobility:** Improved hip mobility resulting from release exercises translates into better functional movement patterns, including walking, running, squatting, and bending, facilitating ease of movement and reducing the risk of injury.

4. Integrating Release for Tight Hips into Somatic Practice:

- **Pre-Workout Preparation:** Incorporate release exercises for tight hips into your pre-workout warm-up routine to prepare the hip muscles and joints for physical activity, optimizing movement quality and reducing the risk of injury.

- **Post-Workout Recovery:** Use release exercises as part of your post-workout cooldown to facilitate recovery, release tension accumulated during exercise, and promote relaxation in the hip muscles and connective tissues.

- **Daily Maintenance:** Incorporate hip release exercises into your daily routine as part of a comprehensive self-care regimen to prevent the buildup of tension and stiffness in the hip region and maintain optimal hip health.

5. Precautions and Considerations:

- **Mindful Approach:** Approach hip release exercises mindfully, paying attention to your body's feedback and avoiding any movements or stretches that cause pain or discomfort.

- **Progress Gradually:** Progress gradually in your hip release practice, increasing the intensity and duration of stretches and mobilization exercises over time as your hip flexibility and mobility improve.

- **Individualized Modification:** Modify hip release exercises to suit your individual needs and abilities, adjusting the range of motion, intensity, and duration of the exercises as necessary to ensure safety and comfort.

6. Advanced Variations of Release for Tight Hips:

- **Proprioceptive Challenges:** Integrate proprioceptive challenges into hip release exercises, such as performing movements on unstable surfaces or incorporating balance exercises, to enhance neuromuscular control and stability in the hip joint.

- **Functional Movement Integration:** Incorporate functional movement patterns into hip release exercises, such as lunges, squats, or hip hinges, to simulate real-life movements and promote greater integration of hip flexibility and mobility into daily activities.

In summary, release exercises for tight hips are indispensable somatic practices for easing hip tension, enhancing flexibility, and promoting better mobility in the hip region. By incorporating hip release into your somatic workout routine and practicing the exercises mindfully and regularly, you can experience significant improvements in hip comfort, mobility, and overall well-being.

Relaxation Sequence: Cultivating Deep Relaxation and Stress Reduction

A relaxation sequence is a vital component of somatic exercises for pain relief, aimed at fostering deep relaxation, reducing stress, and promoting overall well-being. This section delves into the principles, techniques, benefits, and applications of relaxation sequences within the context of somatic practice.

1. Understanding Relaxation Sequences:

- **Overview:** A relaxation sequence consists of a series of somatic exercises and techniques designed to induce a state of deep relaxation in the body and mind.

- **Purpose:** The primary objective of a relaxation sequence is to activate the body's relaxation response, counteracting the effects of stress and tension, and promoting physical, mental, and emotional well-being.

2. Techniques for Performing Relaxation Sequences:

- **Progressive Muscle Relaxation (PMR):** Practice PMR by systematically tensing and releasing each muscle group in the body, starting from the toes and working up to the head, to induce a state of deep relaxation and release tension.

- **Breathwork:** Engage in diaphragmatic breathing techniques, such as belly breathing or paced breathing, to slow down the breath, activate the parasympathetic nervous system, and promote relaxation.

- **Visualization:** Use guided imagery or visualization exercises to mentally transport yourself to a peaceful, tranquil environment, promoting relaxation and reducing stress and anxiety.

- **Body Scan:** Perform a body scan meditation, systematically bringing awareness to each part of the body, from head to toe, and releasing tension and discomfort with each breath, promoting deep relaxation and mindfulness.

3. Benefits of Relaxation Sequences:

- **Stress Reduction:** Relaxation sequences help reduce stress by activating the body's relaxation response, lowering cortisol levels, and promoting a sense of calm and well-being.

- **Muscle Relaxation:** By releasing tension and tightness in the muscles, relaxation sequences alleviate muscular discomfort and promote relaxation throughout the body.

- **Improved Sleep Quality:** Regular practice of relaxation sequences can improve sleep quality by promoting relaxation and reducing the physiological and psychological arousal that interferes with restful sleep.

4. Integrating Relaxation Sequences into Somatic Practice:

- **Daily Practice:** Incorporate relaxation sequences into your daily routine as part of a self-care regimen to reduce stress, promote relaxation, and enhance overall well-being.

- **Pre-Bedtime Routine:** Use relaxation sequences as part of your pre-bedtime routine to unwind, relax, and prepare your body and mind for restful sleep.

- **Stress Management:** Practice relaxation sequences during times of heightened stress or anxiety to promote relaxation, reduce tension, and restore a sense of calm and equilibrium.

5. Precautions and Considerations:

- **Environment:** Create a quiet, comfortable environment free from distractions to practice relaxation sequences, allowing yourself to fully immerse in the experience of relaxation.

- **Patience and Persistence:** Be patient and persistent in your practice of relaxation sequences, recognizing that relaxation is a skill that requires time and practice to develop.

- **Individual Variation:** Modify relaxation techniques to suit your individual preferences and needs, experimenting with different techniques and approaches to find what works best for you.

6. Advanced Variations of Relaxation Sequences:

- **Yoga Nidra:** Explore yoga nidra, also known as yogic sleep, a guided meditation technique that induces deep relaxation and promotes self-awareness and inner peace.

- **Autogenic Training:** Practice autogenic training, a relaxation technique that involves repeating a series of self-directed relaxation phrases to induce a state of deep relaxation and reduce stress and anxiety.

In summary, relaxation sequences are essential somatic practices for cultivating deep relaxation, reducing stress, and promoting overall well-being. By incorporating relaxation sequences into your somatic practice and practicing them mindfully and regularly, you can experience significant improvements in relaxation, stress reduction, and overall quality of life.

Chapter 7

Somatic Exercises for Posture and Alignment

Core Stability: Strengthening the Core Muscles for Better Posture

Core stability exercises play a crucial role in somatic practices for improving posture and alignment. This section explores the principles, techniques, benefits, and applications of core stability exercises within the context of somatic workout.

1. Understanding Core Stability:

- **Overview:** Core stability refers to the ability of the muscles in the trunk and pelvis to maintain optimal alignment and support the spine during movement and weight-bearing activities.

- **Purpose:** The primary aim of core stability exercises is to strengthen the deep stabilizing muscles of the core, including the abdominals, obliques, transverse abdominis, and multifidus, to promote better posture, spinal alignment, and overall movement efficiency.

2. Techniques for Performing Core Stability Exercises:

- **Activation Exercises:** Engage in activation exercises to target the deep core muscles, such as pelvic tilts, abdominal hollowing, and drawing-in maneuvers, to awaken and activate these muscles before engaging in more dynamic movements.

- **Isometric Holds:** Perform isometric holds, such as planks, side planks, and bird-dogs, to challenge and strengthen the core muscles while maintaining a neutral spine and pelvis position.

- **Dynamic Movements:** Incorporate dynamic movements that require core stabilization, such as deadbugs, Russian twists, and mountain climbers, to improve core strength, endurance, and functional stability.

- **Integration with Breathwork:** Coordinate core stability exercises with breathwork techniques, such as synchronized breathing with movement or diaphragmatic breathing during static holds, to enhance coordination, focus, and relaxation.

3. Benefits of Core Stability Exercises:

- **Improved Posture:** Core stability exercises help improve posture by strengthening the muscles that support the spine and pelvis, reducing the risk of slouching, rounding of the shoulders, and excessive arching of the lower back.

- **Enhanced Spinal Alignment:** By promoting better alignment and stability of the spine, core stability exercises help alleviate strain and tension on the spine and surrounding structures, reducing the risk of back pain and injury.

- **Increased Functional Strength:** Strengthening the core muscles through stability exercises enhances overall functional strength and performance in daily activities, sports, and exercise routines.

4. Integrating Core Stability Exercises into Somatic Practice:

- **Foundational Component:** Make core stability exercises a foundational component of your somatic workout routine, performing them regularly to build and maintain core strength and stability.

- **Pre-Workout Activation:** Incorporate core stability exercises into your pre-workout warm-up routine to activate and engage the core muscles, preparing them for more intense physical activity and reducing the risk of injury.

- **Post-Workout Cool Down:** Use core stability exercises as part of your post-workout cooldown to maintain core strength and stability, promote recovery, and restore proper alignment and posture.

5. Precautions and Considerations:

- **Proper Form:** Pay attention to proper form and alignment when performing core stability exercises, maintaining a neutral spine and pelvis position and avoiding excessive arching or rounding of the back.

- **Progression:** Progress gradually in your core stability practice, increasing the intensity and complexity of exercises over time as your core strength and stability improve.

- **Individual Variation:** Modify core stability exercises to suit your individual needs and abilities, adjusting the range of motion, intensity, and duration of exercises as necessary to ensure safety and effectiveness.

6. Advanced Variations of Core Stability Exercises:

- **Unilateral Movements:** Incorporate unilateral movements, such as single-leg squats, lunges, and single-arm planks, to challenge core stability and balance and promote symmetrical strength development.

- **Proprioceptive Challenges:** Integrate proprioceptive challenges, such as performing core stability exercises on unstable surfaces or with eyes closed, to enhance neuromuscular control, coordination, and stability.

In summary, core stability exercises are essential somatic practices for improving posture, alignment, and functional strength. By incorporating core stability exercises into your somatic workout routine and practicing them mindfully and regularly, you can strengthen your core muscles, improve your posture, and enhance overall movement quality and efficiency.

Upper Body Alignment: Improving Shoulder and Upper Back Alignment

Attaining optimal upper body alignment is a cornerstone of somatic practices for enhancing posture and overall alignment. This section delves into the principles, techniques, benefits, and applications of exercises targeting shoulder and upper back alignment within the somatic workout framework.

1. Understanding Upper Body Alignment:

- **Overview:** Upper body alignment encompasses the positioning and movement of the shoulders, upper back, and chest, which significantly impact overall posture and spinal alignment.

- **Purpose:** The primary objective of exercises targeting upper body alignment is to correct imbalances, release tension, and promote proper alignment of the shoulders and upper back, thereby reducing strain and discomfort and fostering improved posture and movement efficiency.

2. Techniques for Improving Shoulder and Upper Back Alignment:

- **Shoulder Retraction and Depression:** Practice shoulder retraction and depression exercises, such as scapular retractions and shoulder blade squeezes, to strengthen the muscles of the upper back and promote proper alignment of the shoulders.

- **Thoracic Extension:** Perform thoracic extension exercises, such as foam roller thoracic extensions and cat-cow stretches, to mobilize and extend the thoracic spine, counteracting the effects of prolonged sitting and slouching.

- **Pectoral Stretching:** Incorporate pectoral stretching exercises, such as doorway stretches and chest openers, to release tension in the chest muscles and improve shoulder mobility and alignment.

- **Postural Awareness:** Cultivate postural awareness throughout the day, paying attention to the alignment of the shoulders and upper back during sitting, standing, and movement, and making conscious adjustments to maintain proper alignment.

3. Benefits of Improving Shoulder and Upper Back Alignment:

- **Pain Reduction:** Correcting shoulder and upper back alignment imbalances can alleviate muscular tension and discomfort in the neck, shoulders, and upper back, reducing the risk of chronic pain and injury.

- **Improved Posture:** By promoting proper alignment of the shoulders and upper back, exercises targeting upper body alignment help improve posture, reducing the appearance of rounded shoulders, forward head posture, and thoracic kyphosis.

- **Enhanced Movement Efficiency:** Optimal shoulder and upper back alignment facilitate more efficient movement patterns, enhancing range of motion, stability, and strength in the upper body and improving overall movement quality.

4. Integrating Exercises for Upper Body Alignment into Somatic Practice:

- **Daily Practice:** Make exercises for upper body alignment a regular part of your somatic workout routine, performing them daily to maintain proper shoulder and upper back alignment and prevent the buildup of tension and discomfort.

- **Pre-Workout Preparation:** Incorporate exercises for upper body alignment into your pre-workout warm-up routine to prepare the shoulders and upper back for movement, reducing the risk of injury and improving exercise performance.

- **Post-Workout Recovery:** Use exercises for upper body alignment as part of your post-workout cooldown to release tension, improve flexibility, and restore proper alignment in the shoulders and upper back, promoting recovery and reducing muscle soreness.

5. Precautions and Considerations:

- **Gradual Progression:** Progress gradually in your practice of exercises for upper body alignment, gradually increasing the intensity and duration of stretches and strengthening exercises over time as your shoulder and upper back mobility and strength improve.

- **Mindful Movement:** Approach exercises for upper body alignment with mindfulness and awareness, paying attention to your body's feedback and avoiding any movements or stretches that cause pain or discomfort.

- **Consistency:** Consistency is key to improving shoulder and upper back alignment. Make a commitment to incorporate exercises for upper body alignment into your daily routine to see lasting improvements in posture and alignment.

6. Advanced Variations of Exercises for Upper Body Alignment:

- **Dynamic Stability Exercises:** Incorporate dynamic stability exercises, such as shoulder stability ball exercises and resistance band rows, to challenge shoulder and upper back alignment while also improving strength and stability.

- **Functional Movement Integration:** Integrate exercises for upper body alignment into functional movement patterns, such as overhead presses, rows, and pulling exercises, to promote better alignment and posture during everyday activities and exercise routines.

In summary, exercises targeting shoulder and upper back alignment are integral components of somatic practices for improving posture and overall alignment. By incorporating these exercises into your somatic workout routine and practicing them mindfully and consistently, you can correct imbalances, release tension, and promote proper alignment of the shoulders and upper back, leading to reduced discomfort, improved posture, and enhanced movement efficiency.

Lower Body Alignment: Enhancing Pelvic Stability and Lower Limb Alignment

In this section, we delve into somatic exercises specifically designed to improve lower body alignment, focusing on enhancing pelvic stability and optimizing lower limb alignment for improved posture and movement efficiency.

1. Understanding Lower Body Alignment:

- **Pelvic Stability:** The pelvis serves as the foundation of the lower body, providing stability and support for the spine and lower limbs. Optimal pelvic alignment is essential for maintaining balance, distributing weight evenly, and preventing strain or injury.

- **Lower Limb Alignment:** Proper alignment of the lower limbs, including the hips, knees, and ankles, is crucial for optimal biomechanics and functional movement. Misalignment in these joints can lead to issues such as hip or knee pain, reduced mobility, and compromised posture.

2. Somatic Exercises for Pelvic Stability:

- **Pelvic Tilts:** Practice pelvic tilting exercises to release tension in the lower back and pelvis while promoting awareness of pelvic positioning. Perform anterior and posterior pelvic tilts while lying on your back, focusing on gently rocking the pelvis forward and backward to find a neutral pelvic position.

- **Hip Circles:** Engage in hip circle movements to mobilize the hip joints and improve pelvic mobility. Stand with feet hip-width apart and gently circle the hips in a clockwise and counterclockwise direction, focusing on fluid, controlled movements to loosen tight hip muscles and promote pelvic stability.

3. Somatic Exercises for Lower Limb Alignment:

- **Hip Hinge:** Practice hip hinge exercises to strengthen the hip extensors and improve hip alignment during movements such as bending and lifting. Stand with feet hip-width apart, hinge at the hips while keeping the spine neutral, and engage the glutes and hamstrings to return to the starting position, focusing on maintaining alignment throughout the movement.

- **Knee Alignment Awareness:** Develop awareness of knee alignment during weight-bearing activities such as walking, squatting, or lunging. Pay attention to the alignment of the knees relative to the feet and hips, ensuring that they track in line with the toes and do not collapse inward or outward, which can place undue stress on the knee joints.

4. Integrating Breath and Movement:

- **Diaphragmatic Breathing:** Incorporate diaphragmatic breathing techniques into somatic exercises for lower body alignment to enhance relaxation, reduce tension, and promote core stability. Practice deep, rhythmic breathing while performing pelvic stability and lower limb alignment exercises, allowing the breath to facilitate movement and support alignment.

5. Mindful Movement Practices:

- **Body Scanning:** Utilize body scanning techniques to enhance proprioception and body awareness during somatic exercises for lower body alignment. Scan through the pelvis, hips, knees, and ankles, noting any areas of tension or misalignment, and use breath awareness and gentle movement to release tension and restore balance.

6. Benefits of Lower Body Alignment Exercises:

- **Improved Posture:** Somatic exercises for lower body alignment help correct imbalances and misalignments, promoting optimal posture and spinal alignment.

- **Reduced Risk of Injury:** By enhancing pelvic stability and lower limb alignment, these exercises reduce the risk of strain, injury, and wear and tear on the musculoskeletal system during daily activities and physical exertion.

- **Enhanced Movement Efficiency:** Proper alignment of the lower body facilitates efficient movement patterns, allowing for smoother, more coordinated movement and greater ease of mobility in activities of daily living.

In summary, somatic exercises for lower body alignment focus on enhancing pelvic stability and optimizing lower limb alignment to promote optimal posture, movement efficiency, and overall musculoskeletal health. By incorporating these exercises into your regular somatic practice, you can cultivate greater awareness, stability, and balance in the lower body, supporting improved posture and movement quality in everyday life.

Whole-Body Integration: Bringing Balance and Harmony to the Body

Whole-body integration exercises are fundamental in somatic practices for achieving balanced posture and alignment. This section explores the principles, techniques, benefits, and applications of exercises focused on integrating the entire body within the somatic workout framework.

1. Understanding Whole-Body Integration:

- **Overview:** Whole-body integration involves connecting and coordinating movement patterns throughout the entire body to achieve balanced posture and alignment.

- **Purpose:** The primary objective of whole-body integration exercises is to promote harmony and synergy among different muscle groups and joints, fostering improved movement efficiency, balance, and overall body awareness.

2. Techniques for Whole-Body Integration:

- **Functional Movement Patterns:** Engage in functional movement patterns that involve coordinated movements of multiple joints and muscle groups, such as squats, lunges, and rotational movements, to promote whole-body integration and improve movement quality.

- **Dynamic Stability Exercises:** Perform dynamic stability exercises, such as single-leg movements, balance exercises, and proprioceptive drills, to challenge and improve neuromuscular control and coordination throughout the body.

- **Flowing Movement Sequences:** Practice flowing movement sequences that seamlessly transition between different exercises and movement patterns, such as yoga flows, tai chi forms, and dance-inspired movements, to promote fluidity and integration in movement.

- **Breathwork Integration:** Coordinate movement with breathwork techniques, such as linking specific movements with inhalation and exhalation patterns, to enhance relaxation, focus, and body awareness during whole-body integration exercises.

3. Benefits of Whole-Body Integration:

- **Improved Movement Quality:** Whole-body integration exercises enhance movement quality by promoting coordination, balance, and fluidity in movement patterns, reducing the risk of injury and improving overall movement efficiency.

- **Enhanced Body Awareness:** By connecting and coordinating movements throughout the entire body, whole-body integration exercises cultivate greater body awareness and proprioception, facilitating improved posture, alignment, and movement control.

- **Stress Reduction:** Engaging in whole-body integration exercises can reduce stress and tension in the body and mind, promoting relaxation, mental clarity, and a sense of well-being.

4. Integrating Whole-Body Integration Exercises into Somatic Practice:

- **Holistic Approach:** Embrace a holistic approach to movement by incorporating whole-body integration exercises into your somatic workout routine, focusing on connecting and coordinating movements throughout the entire body.

- **Mind-Body Connection:** Cultivate a strong mind-body connection during whole-body integration exercises, paying attention to sensations, alignment, and movement quality, and making adjustments as needed to promote balance and harmony.

- **Variety and Creativity:** Explore a variety of whole-body integration exercises and movement modalities, incorporating creativity and experimentation to keep your practice engaging and enjoyable.

5. Precautions and Considerations:

- **Listen to Your Body:** Pay attention to your body's signals during whole-body integration exercises, respecting your limits and avoiding any movements or positions that cause pain or discomfort.

- **Progression:** Progress gradually in your practice of whole-body integration exercises, starting with simpler movements and gradually increasing the complexity and intensity of exercises as your movement skills and body awareness improve.

- **Rest and Recovery:** Allow for adequate rest and recovery between whole-body integration sessions, giving your body time to adapt and recover from the demands of movement practice.

6. Advanced Variations of Whole-Body Integration Exercises:

- **Mindful Movement Challenges:** Integrate mindfulness challenges into whole-body integration exercises, such as performing movements with eyes closed or focusing on subtle sensations and nuances of movement, to enhance body awareness and concentration.

- **Integrative Movement Modalities:** Explore integrative movement modalities that combine different movement disciplines, such as martial arts, gymnastics, and dance, to promote holistic development of movement skills and body awareness.

In summary, whole-body integration exercises are essential components of somatic practices for improving posture, alignment, and movement quality. By incorporating these exercises into your somatic workout routine and practicing them mindfully and consistently, you can cultivate balanced movement patterns, enhance body awareness, and promote harmony and synergy throughout the entire body.

Chapter 8

Advanced Practices and Progressions

Incorporating Somatic Movement into Other Forms of Exercise

Integrating somatic movement into other forms of exercise represents an advanced practice that can enhance the effectiveness, safety, and enjoyment of various physical activities. This section delves into the principles, techniques, benefits, and applications of incorporating somatic movement into different exercise modalities.

1. Understanding Integration of Somatic Movement:

- **Overview:** Integrating somatic movement into other forms of exercise involves blending somatic principles and techniques with existing exercise modalities to enhance movement quality, efficiency, and mind-body connection.

- **Purpose:** The primary objective of incorporating somatic movement into other forms of exercise is to optimize movement patterns, improve body awareness, and reduce the risk of injury while enhancing the overall effectiveness and enjoyment of physical activity.

2. Techniques for Incorporating Somatic Movement:

- **Mindful Movement:** Practice mindful movement techniques during other forms of exercise, such as yoga, Pilates, strength training, or cardiovascular exercise, focusing on body awareness, breath control, and movement quality.

- **Sensory Awareness:** Cultivate sensory awareness during exercise by paying attention to sensations, proprioception, and alignment, and making adjustments to movement patterns to promote optimal movement efficiency and reduce strain.

- **Dynamic Warm-Up:** Incorporate somatic movement exercises into your warm-up routine before engaging in other forms of exercise to prepare the body and mind for movement, enhance mobility, and activate stabilizing muscles.

- **Cool-Down and Recovery:** Use somatic movement exercises as part of your cool-down and recovery routine after exercise to promote relaxation, release tension, and facilitate recovery in the muscles and joints.

3. Benefits of Incorporating Somatic Movement:

- **Enhanced Movement Quality:** Integrating somatic movement into other forms of exercise improves movement quality by promoting better alignment, posture, and body awareness, leading to more efficient and effective movement patterns.

- **Injury Prevention:** By emphasizing proper alignment, movement mechanics, and body awareness, incorporating somatic movement into other forms of exercise helps reduce the risk of injury and overuse by minimizing strain and compensatory movements.

- **Mind-Body Connection:** Practicing somatic movement within other exercise modalities fosters a stronger mind-body connection, enhancing proprioception, concentration, and mindfulness during physical activity.

4. Integrating Somatic Movement into Various Exercise Modalities:

- **Yoga:** Infuse somatic movement principles into yoga practice by focusing on breath awareness, mindful movement, and alignment cues to deepen the mind-body connection and enhance the therapeutic benefits of yoga.

- **Pilates:** Incorporate somatic movement techniques, such as pelvic tilts, spinal articulation, and breathwork, into Pilates exercises to improve core stability, spinal mobility, and overall movement efficiency.

- **Strength Training:** Integrate somatic movement into strength training workouts by emphasizing proper alignment, muscle engagement, and movement quality during exercises such as squats, deadlifts, and rows to enhance muscle activation and reduce the risk of injury.

- **Cardiovascular Exercise:** Apply somatic movement principles to cardiovascular workouts, such as running, cycling, or swimming, by focusing on relaxation, efficient movement patterns, and breath control to improve endurance, performance, and overall well-being.

5. Precautions and Considerations:

- **Individualized Approach:** Tailor the integration of somatic movement into other forms of exercise to suit individual needs, preferences, and fitness levels, adjusting the intensity, duration, and complexity of exercises as necessary.

- **Progression:** Progress gradually when incorporating somatic movement into other exercise modalities, starting with simpler techniques and gradually increasing the complexity and integration of somatic principles into your workouts.

- **Consultation:** Consult with a qualified fitness professional or somatic movement instructor to ensure that the integration of somatic movement into other forms of exercise is appropriate for your goals, needs, and physical condition.

6. Advanced Progressions in Integrating Somatic Movement:

- **Advanced Movement Variations:** Explore advanced variations of somatic movement exercises within other exercise modalities, incorporating challenging movement patterns, transitions, and sequences to further enhance movement quality and body awareness.

- **Cross-Training Integration:** Integrate somatic movement into cross-training activities, such as functional fitness, martial arts, or dance, to diversify movement patterns, improve movement efficiency, and enhance overall physical performance.

In summary, incorporating somatic movement into other forms of exercise represents an advanced practice that can enhance movement quality, reduce the risk of injury, and deepen the mind-body connection during physical activity. By integrating somatic principles and techniques into various exercise modalities mindfully and consistently, you can optimize movement patterns, improve body awareness, and enhance overall well-being.

Exploring Movement Variations and Progressions

Delving into advanced movement variations and progressions adds depth and challenge to your somatic practice. This section explores the principles, techniques, benefits, and applications of advancing your movement repertoire within the somatic workout framework.

1. Understanding Advanced Movement Variations:

- **Overview:** Advanced movement variations involve exploring complex and nuanced movement patterns that challenge coordination, strength, and body awareness.

- **Purpose:** The primary objective of advanced movement variations is to deepen your understanding of movement potential, enhance physical capabilities, and foster continuous growth and development in your somatic practice.

2. Techniques for Exploring Movement Variations:

- **Dynamic Movement Sequences:** Create dynamic movement sequences that seamlessly transition between different exercises and movement patterns, incorporating flowing transitions, intricate footwork, and multidirectional movement.

- **Multi-Planar Movements:** Explore movements in multiple planes of motion, including sagittal, frontal, and transverse planes, to challenge stability, coordination, and proprioception across different movement patterns.

- **Unilateral Movements:** Incorporate unilateral movements, such as single-leg squats, lunges, and unilateral loaded exercises, to challenge balance, stability, and strength asymmetries between the left and right sides of the body.

- **Integration of Props:** Use props such as resistance bands, stability balls, foam rollers, and balance boards to add resistance, instability, and variability to your movement practice, enhancing the challenge and effectiveness of advanced movement variations.

3. Benefits of Exploring Movement Variations:

- **Movement Diversity:** Exploring advanced movement variations introduces diversity and complexity into your movement practice, stimulating adaptation and growth in neuromuscular coordination, strength, and mobility.

- **Skill Development:** Advanced movement variations enhance motor learning and skill development by challenging movement patterns that require precision, timing, and coordination, leading to improved movement efficiency and performance.

- **Mind-Body Integration:** Engaging in advanced movement variations fosters a deeper mind-body connection, requiring heightened body awareness, concentration, and focus to execute complex movement sequences with fluidity and control.

4. Progressions in Movement Variations:

- **Gradual Complexity:** Progress gradually in exploring movement variations, starting with simpler variations and gradually increasing the complexity and challenge of movement patterns as your skills and capabilities develop.

- **Incremental Load:** Introduce incremental load and intensity to movement variations by gradually increasing resistance, speed, range of motion, or duration of exercises to stimulate adaptation and progression in strength and conditioning.

- **Mindful Practice:** Approach advanced movement variations with mindfulness and awareness, paying attention to movement quality, alignment, and sensations, and making adjustments as needed to maintain proper form and technique.

5. Integrating Movement Variations into Somatic Practice:

- **Creative Exploration:** Embrace creativity and exploration in your somatic practice by experimenting with different movement variations, improvising sequences, and combining elements from various movement disciplines.

- **Functional Application:** Consider the functional application of movement variations to everyday activities, sports, and exercise routines, focusing on movements that translate into improved performance and functionality in daily life.

- **Playful Spirit:** Maintain a playful and curious spirit in your exploration of movement variations, approaching each practice session with a sense of openness, curiosity, and joy in movement discovery.

6. Precautions and Considerations:

- **Respect Individual Limits:** Respect your individual limits and capabilities when exploring advanced movement variations, avoiding pushing beyond your current skill level or risking injury.

- **Consultation:** Consult with a qualified fitness professional or somatic movement instructor to ensure that the exploration of advanced movement variations is appropriate for your goals, needs, and physical condition.

- **Progression Monitoring:** Monitor your progression in exploring movement variations, paying attention to improvements in movement quality, strength, and mobility, and adjusting your practice accordingly to continue challenging yourself effectively.

7. Advanced Variations of Movement Progressions:

- **Combination Movements:** Combine different movement patterns and modalities, such as yoga poses with strength training exercises or martial arts techniques with dance movements, to create unique and challenging movement sequences.

- **Environmental Challenges:** Integrate environmental challenges into your movement practice, such as practicing outdoors on uneven terrain or incorporating natural obstacles like rocks, trees, or hills, to add variability and unpredictability to your movement experience.

In summary, exploring advanced movement variations and progressions adds richness, depth, and challenge to your somatic practice, fostering continuous growth and development in movement capabilities, body awareness, and overall well-being. By embracing creativity, curiosity, and mindfulness in your exploration of movement variations, you can unlock new levels of skill, proficiency, and joy in movement discovery.

Somatic Flow Sequences: Connecting Movements in Fluid Sequences

Somatic flow sequences represent an advanced practice within somatic movement, emphasizing the seamless integration of movements into fluid and continuous sequences. This section explores the principles, techniques, benefits, and applications of somatic flow sequences within the somatic workout framework.

1. Understanding Somatic Flow Sequences:

- **Overview:** Somatic flow sequences involve linking movements together in a fluid and continuous manner, emphasizing smooth transitions, breath coordination, and mindful awareness throughout the sequence.

- **Purpose:** The primary objective of somatic flow sequences is to cultivate a sense of flow, rhythm, and integration in movement, promoting enhanced body awareness, coordination, and mindfulness.

2. Techniques for Creating Somatic Flow Sequences:

- **Breath Synchronization:** Coordinate movements with breath patterns, using inhalation and exhalation to guide the rhythm and timing of the sequence, promoting relaxation, focus, and embodiment.

- **Seamless Transitions:** Focus on creating seamless transitions between movements, minimizing pauses and interruptions to maintain the flow and continuity of the sequence, fostering a sense of fluidity and integration in movement.

- **Mindful Awareness:** Cultivate mindful awareness throughout the sequence, paying attention to sensations, alignment, and movement quality, and making subtle adjustments as needed to maintain optimal body mechanics and alignment.

- **Creative Expression:** Embrace creativity and spontaneity in designing somatic flow sequences, allowing for exploration and experimentation with different movement patterns, variations, and modalities.

3. Benefits of Somatic Flow Sequences:

- **Enhanced Body Awareness:** Somatic flow sequences deepen body awareness by encouraging mindful attention to sensations, movement quality, and breath, fostering a deeper connection to the body and its innate intelligence.

- **Improved Coordination:** By emphasizing smooth transitions and rhythmic movement patterns, somatic flow sequences enhance coordination, timing, and spatial awareness, promoting more efficient and graceful movement.

- **Stress Reduction:** Engaging in somatic flow sequences promotes relaxation, stress reduction, and mental clarity by facilitating a state of flow and presence in movement, helping to alleviate tension and anxiety.

4. Applications of Somatic Flow Sequences:

- **Personal Practice:** Incorporate somatic flow sequences into your personal movement practice as a means of self-expression, exploration, and self-discovery, allowing for a creative and embodied exploration of movement.

- **Group Classes:** Lead or participate in group somatic flow classes, where participants move together in synchrony, exploring movement variations and improvisation within the context of a supportive and collaborative environment.

- **Therapeutic Settings:** Utilize somatic flow sequences in therapeutic settings, such as rehabilitation or stress management programs, to facilitate movement exploration, body awareness, and emotional integration.

5. Precautions and Considerations:

- **Respect Individual Limits:** Respect your individual limits and capabilities when practicing somatic flow sequences, listening to your body's signals and avoiding pushing beyond your current comfort level or risking injury.

- **Progression:** Progress gradually in your practice of somatic flow sequences, starting with simpler sequences and gradually increasing the complexity and intensity of movements as your skills and body awareness develop.

- **Mindful Practice:** Approach somatic flow sequences with mindfulness and awareness, focusing on the quality of movement, breath coordination, and embodied presence throughout the sequence.

6. Advanced Variations of Somatic Flow Sequences:

- **Theme-Based Sequences:** Create theme-based somatic flow sequences, focusing on specific movement qualities, intentions, or areas of focus, such as balance, flexibility, or emotional expression, to deepen the exploration and embodiment of movement.

- **Prop Integration:** Incorporate props such as yoga blocks, straps, or balls into somatic flow sequences to add variety, challenge, and creativity to the practice, encouraging exploration and playfulness in movement.

In summary, somatic flow sequences offer a dynamic and expressive approach to movement practice, emphasizing fluidity, mindfulness, and embodied presence. By incorporating somatic flow sequences into your somatic workout routine and practicing them with awareness and intention, you can cultivate enhanced body awareness, coordination, and relaxation while fostering a deeper connection to yourself and your movement experience.

Partner and Group Somatic Practices: Enhancing Connection and Community

Partner and group somatic practices represent an advanced level of engagement within somatic movement, focusing on interpersonal connection, mutual support, and shared embodiment experiences. This section explores the principles, techniques, benefits, and applications of partner and group somatic practices within the somatic workout framework.

1. Understanding Partner and Group Somatic Practices:

- **Overview:** Partner and group somatic practices involve engaging in somatic movement exercises and explorations with one or more partners or within a group setting.

- **Purpose:** The primary objective of partner and group somatic practices is to cultivate interpersonal connection, mutual support, and shared embodiment experiences, fostering a sense of community and collective presence in movement.

2. Techniques for Partner and Group Somatic Practices:

- **Partner Movement Exploration:** Engage in partnered movement explorations, such as mirroring exercises, contact improvisation, or shared weight-bearing exercises, to cultivate non-verbal communication, trust, and connection with your partner.

- **Group Movement Dynamics:** Participate in group movement dynamics, such as synchronized movement sequences, collective improvisation, or group breathwork exercises, to experience the interconnectedness and synergy of group embodiment.

- **Partner Assisted Stretching:** Explore partner-assisted stretching techniques, such as reciprocal inhibition stretching or proprioceptive neuromuscular facilitation (PNF), to deepen stretches and release tension with the support of a partner.

- **Group Meditation and Mindfulness:** Practice group meditation and mindfulness exercises, such as guided body scans, mindful movement meditations, or group breathwork sessions, to cultivate collective presence, relaxation, and inner awareness within the group.

3. Benefits of Partner and Group Somatic Practices:

- **Enhanced Connection:** Partner and group somatic practices foster enhanced interpersonal connection, communication, and empathy through shared movement experiences and embodied presence.

- **Mutual Support:** Engaging in partner and group somatic practices provides opportunities for mutual support, encouragement, and collaboration, creating a supportive and nurturing environment for personal growth and exploration.

- **Sense of Community:** Participating in partner and group somatic practices cultivates a sense of community and belonging, fostering a shared sense of purpose, identity, and connection among group members.

4. Applications of Partner and Group Somatic Practices:

- **Workshops and Retreats:** Attend somatic movement workshops, retreats, or group classes that focus on partner and group somatic practices, offering opportunities for deep exploration, connection, and community building within a supportive and immersive environment.

- **Therapeutic Settings:** Utilize partner and group somatic practices in therapeutic settings, such as group therapy sessions, trauma-informed yoga classes, or body-based psychotherapy groups, to facilitate interpersonal connection, emotional expression, and healing within the group context.

- **Team Building and Leadership Development:** Incorporate partner and group somatic practices into team-building workshops, leadership development programs, or corporate wellness initiatives, offering opportunities for team bonding, communication skills development, and stress reduction within organizational settings.

5. Precautions and Considerations:

- **Respect Boundaries:** Respect personal boundaries and comfort levels when engaging in partner and group somatic practices, allowing individuals to opt out of specific activities or adjustments if they feel uncomfortable or unsafe.

- **Clear Communication:** Foster clear and open communication within partner and group somatic practices, encouraging participants to express their needs, preferences, and boundaries openly and respectfully.

- **Inclusivity:** Ensure inclusivity and accessibility within partner and group somatic practices, creating a welcoming and inclusive environment that honors diversity of backgrounds, experiences, and identities.

6. Advanced Variations of Partner and Group Somatic Practices:

- **Shared Leadership:** Explore shared leadership models within partner and group somatic practices, empowering participants to take turns leading exercises, facilitating discussions, or guiding movement explorations, fostering a sense of co-creation and empowerment within the group.

- **Community Rituals and Ceremonies:** Create community rituals and ceremonies within partner and group somatic practices, such as group circles, sharing circles, or collective movement rituals, to honor transitions, celebrate milestones, or cultivate intentionality and meaning within the group context.

In summary, partner and group somatic practices offer unique opportunities for interpersonal connection, mutual support, and shared embodiment experiences within the somatic movement community. By engaging in partner and group somatic practices with mindfulness, empathy, and openness, participants can deepen their connection to themselves, each other, and the collective wisdom of the group, fostering a sense of belonging, connection, and community in movement exploration and embodiment.

Chapter 9

Somatic Workout for Everyday Life

Incorporating Somatic Principles into Daily Activities

Incorporating somatic principles into daily activities extends the benefits of somatic practice beyond dedicated workout sessions, promoting mindfulness, body awareness, and movement efficiency in everyday life. This section explores the principles, techniques, benefits, and applications of integrating somatic principles into various daily activities within the somatic workout framework.

1. Understanding Somatic Principles in Daily Activities:

- **Overview:** Somatic principles emphasize mindful awareness, movement efficiency, and body-mind integration, which can be applied to a wide range of daily activities, from sitting and standing to walking and lifting.

- **Purpose:** The primary objective of incorporating somatic principles into daily activities is to promote enhanced body awareness, movement quality, and well-being throughout the day, fostering mindfulness and presence in everyday life.

2. Techniques for Incorporating Somatic Principles:

- **Mindful Movement:** Practice mindful movement during daily activities, paying attention to body sensations, alignment, and breath, and making conscious adjustments to promote optimal movement mechanics and efficiency.

- **Body Scan:** Incorporate brief body scan exercises into daily routines, taking moments to scan the body for areas of tension, discomfort, or imbalance, and using breath and awareness to release tension and promote relaxation.

- **Postural Awareness:** Cultivate postural awareness throughout the day, paying attention to alignment and posture during sitting, standing, walking, and other activities, and making subtle adjustments to promote optimal spinal alignment and muscular balance.

- **Movement Variability:** Embrace movement variability in daily activities, exploring different movement patterns, positions, and ranges of motion to prevent stiffness, promote joint health, and improve movement efficiency.

3. Benefits of Incorporating Somatic Principles into Daily Activities:

- **Improved Body Awareness:** By applying somatic principles to daily activities, individuals develop greater body awareness, sensitivity, and responsiveness to internal cues and external stimuli, promoting a deeper connection to the body and its needs.

- **Enhanced Movement Quality:** Integrating somatic principles into daily activities enhances movement quality, efficiency, and coordination, reducing the risk of strain, injury, and discomfort while promoting ease, grace, and fluidity in movement.

- **Stress Reduction:** Engaging mindfully in daily activities with somatic awareness promotes relaxation, stress reduction, and mental clarity, helping individuals navigate daily challenges with greater resilience, presence, and calm.

4. Applications of Somatic Principles in Daily Activities:

- **Sitting and Standing:** Practice mindful sitting and standing by paying attention to spinal alignment, weight distribution, and muscular engagement, using breath and awareness to release tension and promote ease in static postures.

- **Walking and Movement:** Incorporate somatic principles into walking and movement patterns by focusing on foot placement, hip mobility, and arm swing, and cultivating a sense of groundedness, balance, and flow in movement.

- **Lifting and Carrying:** Apply somatic principles to lifting and carrying objects by engaging core stability, hip hinge mechanics, and proper lifting technique, minimizing strain and risk of injury while promoting efficient and safe movement.

- **Computer and Screen Use:** Utilize somatic principles during computer and screen use by taking regular movement breaks, practicing eye relaxation exercises, and maintaining ergonomic alignment to prevent discomfort and fatigue.

5. Precautions and Considerations:

- **Gradual Integration:** Gradually integrate somatic principles into daily activities, starting with small, manageable changes and gradually expanding awareness and mindfulness to more activities and situations over time.

- **Patience and Persistence:** Be patient and persistent in applying somatic principles to daily activities, recognizing that change takes time and consistency, and embracing the process of learning and growth.

- **Self-Compassion:** Cultivate self-compassion and kindness towards yourself as you navigate the challenges and successes of integrating somatic principles into daily life, acknowledging that each moment presents an opportunity for learning and growth.

6. Advanced Variations of Incorporating Somatic Principles:

- **Multitasking Mindfulness:** Practice multitasking mindfulness by applying somatic principles to everyday activities that involve simultaneous physical and mental engagement, such as cooking, cleaning, or commuting, fostering presence and awareness amidst daily busyness.

- **Environmental Adaptation:** Adapt somatic principles to different environments and contexts, such as home, work, or travel, finding creative ways to integrate mindfulness, movement, and embodiment into diverse daily routines and lifestyles.

In summary, incorporating somatic principles into daily activities offers a practical and accessible way to promote mindfulness, body awareness, and movement efficiency in everyday life. By applying somatic principles to sitting, standing, walking, lifting, and other daily activities with mindfulness and intention, individuals can enhance their overall well-being, resilience, and quality of life.

Somatic Practices for Stress Management and Emotional Well-Being

Somatic practices offer valuable tools for managing stress, cultivating emotional resilience, and promoting overall well-being in daily life. This section explores various somatic techniques and exercises specifically tailored to support stress management and emotional balance within the context of everyday activities.

1. Understanding Somatic Practices for Stress Management:

- **Overview:** Somatic practices for stress management focus on using movement, breath, and body awareness to regulate the nervous system, release tension, and promote relaxation in response to stressors encountered in daily life.

- **Purpose:** The primary objective of somatic practices for stress management is to cultivate greater resilience, emotional regulation, and well-being by fostering a deeper connection to the body and its innate capacity for self-regulation and healing.

2. Techniques for Somatic Stress Management:

- **Breath Awareness:** Practice conscious breathing exercises, such as diaphragmatic breathing or mindful breathing, to regulate the autonomic nervous system, promote relaxation, and reduce the physiological effects of stress on the body.

- **Gentle Movement:** Engage in gentle somatic movement practices, such as slow, mindful stretching or flowing movement sequences, to release muscular tension, increase body awareness, and promote a sense of ease and relaxation.

- **Body Scan Meditation:** Practice body scan meditation, systematically scanning the body for areas of tension or discomfort and using breath and awareness to release tension and promote relaxation from head to toe.

- **Grounding Techniques:** Utilize grounding techniques, such as mindful walking, barefoot grounding, or body awareness exercises, to anchor attention in the present moment, connect with the earth, and foster a sense of stability and security amidst stressors.

3. Benefits of Somatic Practices for Stress Management:

- **Stress Reduction:** Somatic practices for stress management promote relaxation, reduce physiological arousal, and mitigate the effects of chronic stress on the body and mind, fostering a greater sense of calm, balance, and well-being.

- **Emotional Regulation:** By cultivating body awareness and mindful presence, somatic practices support emotional regulation and resilience, helping individuals navigate challenging emotions with greater equanimity, clarity, and self-compassion.

- **Enhanced Resilience:** Regular practice of somatic techniques for stress management strengthens the resilience of the nervous system, increasing capacity to cope with adversity, adapt to change, and bounce back from challenging situations.

4. Applications of Somatic Practices for Stress Management:

- **Daily Stress Reduction:** Integrate brief somatic practices into daily routines, such as morning rituals, work breaks, or bedtime routines, to proactively manage stress and promote emotional well-being throughout the day.

- **Stressful Situations:** Use somatic techniques to cope with acute stressors or challenging situations, such as deadlines, conflicts, or unexpected events, by engaging in grounding practices, breath awareness, or gentle movement to regulate stress responses and restore equilibrium.

- **Self-Care Practices:** Incorporate somatic practices into self-care routines, such as relaxation baths, self-massage, or restorative yoga, to nurture physical, mental, and emotional well-being and replenish vital energy reserves.

5. Precautions and Considerations:

- **Individualized Approach:** Tailor somatic practices for stress management to suit individual preferences, needs, and abilities, respecting personal boundaries and comfort levels when exploring new techniques or exercises.

- **Consistency:** Cultivate a consistent somatic practice for stress management, integrating techniques into daily life with regularity and commitment to maximize effectiveness and long-term benefits.

- **Professional Guidance:** Seek guidance from a qualified somatic practitioner, therapist, or healthcare provider when navigating complex or persistent stress-related issues, ensuring appropriate support and guidance in addressing underlying causes and promoting holistic well-being.

6. Advanced Variations of Somatic Stress Management Practices:

- **Trauma-Informed Practices:** Explore trauma-informed somatic practices, such as trauma-sensitive yoga or somatic experiencing, to address deeper layers of stress, trauma, or emotional distress with sensitivity, compassion, and skill.

- **Mindfulness-Based Stress Reduction (MBSR):** Participate in structured mindfulness-based stress reduction programs, incorporating somatic practices alongside mindfulness meditation, cognitive strategies, and group support to cultivate resilience and well-being in the face of stress and adversity.

In summary, somatic practices offer valuable tools for managing stress, promoting emotional well-being, and fostering resilience in everyday life. By integrating somatic techniques and exercises into daily routines with mindfulness and intention, individuals can cultivate greater self-awareness, regulate stress responses, and enhance overall quality of life.

Somatic Techniques for Improving Sleep Quality and Relaxation

In today's fast-paced world, stress and tension can often interfere with our ability to relax and achieve restful sleep. This section explores various somatic techniques tailored to promote relaxation and enhance sleep quality, fostering overall well-being in daily life.

1. Understanding the Importance of Sleep Quality and Relaxation:

- **Overview:** Quality sleep and relaxation are essential for physical health, mental well-being, and overall vitality. Adequate rest allows the body to repair, rejuvenate, and restore balance, while relaxation promotes stress reduction and emotional resilience.

- **Purpose:** The primary objective of somatic techniques for sleep quality and relaxation is to facilitate the body's natural relaxation response, promoting restful sleep and deep relaxation to support optimal health and well-being.

2. Techniques for Improving Sleep Quality:

- **Breath Awareness:** Practice mindful breathing exercises before bedtime to calm the nervous system, regulate breathing patterns, and prepare the body for sleep. Focus on slow, deep breaths, allowing the breath to become smooth and rhythmic.

- **Progressive Muscle Relaxation (PMR):** Engage in progressive muscle relaxation techniques to release tension and promote relaxation throughout the body. Start by tensing and then slowly releasing each muscle group, from head to toe, to induce a state of deep relaxation conducive to sleep.

- **Body Scan Meditation:** Practice body scan meditation while lying in bed, systematically scanning the body for areas of tension or discomfort. Use breath awareness to gently release tension and promote relaxation, allowing the body to unwind and prepare for sleep.

- **Somatic Movement:** Incorporate gentle somatic movement practices, such as slow, mindful stretching or gentle yoga poses, to release muscular tension, increase body awareness, and promote relaxation before bedtime.

3. Techniques for Enhancing Relaxation:

- **Mindful Movement:** Engage in mindful movement practices, such as tai chi, qigong, or walking meditation, to cultivate present-moment awareness and promote relaxation throughout the body and mind.

- **Breathwork:** Explore different breathwork techniques, such as diaphragmatic breathing, alternate nostril breathing, or square breathing, to regulate the autonomic nervous system, reduce stress, and promote relaxation.

- **Guided Imagery:** Use guided imagery or visualization exercises to create a sense of calm and relaxation. Imagine yourself in a peaceful, serene environment, focusing on sensory details to evoke feelings of relaxation and tranquillity.

- **Self-Massage:** Practice self-massage techniques, such as gentle rubbing or kneading of tense muscles, to promote relaxation and release tension throughout the body.

4. Benefits of Somatic Techniques for Sleep and Relaxation:

- **Improved Sleep Quality:** Somatic techniques promote relaxation and stress reduction, helping to improve sleep quality by facilitating the transition into restful sleep and reducing sleep disturbances.

- **Stress Reduction:** Regular practice of somatic techniques reduces physiological arousal and lowers stress levels, promoting emotional resilience and well-being in daily life.

- **Enhanced Relaxation Response:** Somatic techniques activate the body's relaxation response, triggering physiological changes that promote deep relaxation, reduce muscle tension, and alleviate symptoms of stress and anxiety.

5. Applications of Somatic Techniques in Everyday Life:

- **Bedtime Routine:** Incorporate somatic techniques into your bedtime routine to promote relaxation and prepare the body and mind for sleep. Establish a calming pre-sleep ritual that includes practices such as breathwork, meditation, or gentle movement to signal to the body that it is time to unwind.

- **Stress Management:** Use somatic techniques throughout the day to manage stress and promote relaxation in response to daily stressors. Take short breaks to engage in deep breathing, body scans, or gentle stretching to release tension and restore balance.

- **Relaxation Practices:** Integrate somatic relaxation practices into your daily life to foster a greater sense of calm and well-being. Set aside dedicated time each day for relaxation exercises, such as guided meditation, progressive muscle relaxation, or gentle movement, to promote relaxation and rejuvenation.

6. Precautions and Considerations:

- **Individualized Approach:** Tailor somatic techniques to suit your individual needs, preferences, and limitations. Pay attention to your body's signals and adjust practices accordingly to ensure safety and comfort.

- **Consistency:** Cultivate a consistent somatic practice for sleep and relaxation, incorporating techniques into your daily routine with regularity and commitment to maximize effectiveness and long-term benefits.

- **Professional Guidance:** Seek guidance from qualified somatic practitioners, therapists, or healthcare providers if you experience persistent sleep disturbances or high levels of stress, ensuring appropriate support and guidance in addressing underlying issues and promoting holistic well-being.

In summary, somatic techniques offer valuable tools for improving sleep quality and promoting relaxation in everyday life. By incorporating breath awareness, mindful movement, guided meditation, and other somatic practices into your daily routine, you can cultivate a greater sense of calm, balance, and well-being, enhancing overall health and vitality.

Cultivating a Somatic Mind-set: Living Mindfully in Every Moment

Living with a somatic mind-set involves embodying mindfulness, awareness, and presence in every aspect of daily life. This section explores the principles, techniques, benefits, and applications of cultivating a somatic mind-set to enhance overall well-being and fulfilment in everyday life.

1. Understanding the Somatic mind-set:

- **Overview:** The somatic mind-set emphasizes the cultivation of mindfulness, body awareness, and presence in daily life, anchoring attention in the present moment and fostering a deeper connection to the body's innate wisdom and intelligence.

- **Purpose:** The primary objective of cultivating a somatic mind-set is to promote greater awareness, authenticity, and vitality in everyday experiences, enhancing overall well-being and quality of life.

2. Techniques for Cultivating a Somatic mind-set:

- **Embodied Presence:** Practice embodied presence by anchoring attention in physical sensations, such as breath, movement, or tactile sensations, and cultivating awareness of bodily sensations as a gateway to present-moment experience.

- **Sensory Awareness:** Cultivate sensory awareness by engaging all five senses—sight, hearing, touch, taste, and smell—in everyday activities, savoring sensory experiences with curiosity, openness, and receptivity.

- **Mindful Movement:** Incorporate mindful movement into daily routines, such as walking mindfully, eating mindfully, or performing daily tasks with awareness and intention, fostering a deeper connection to the body and its inherent wisdom.

- **Body-Mind Integration:** Explore the interconnectedness of body and mind by noticing the impact of thoughts, emotions, and beliefs on bodily sensations and vice versa, recognizing the intimate relationship between mental and physical well-being.

3. Benefits of a Somatic mind-set:

- **Enhanced Awareness:** Cultivating a somatic mind-set enhances overall awareness of internal and external experiences, promoting clarity, insight, and discernment in navigating life's challenges and opportunities.

- **Authentic Expression:** Living with a somatic mind-set encourages authentic self-expression and embodiment, allowing individuals to honour their unique needs, preferences, and values with greater integrity and authenticity.

- **Vitality and Fulfilment:** By anchoring attention in the present moment and embracing life with openness and curiosity, a somatic mind-set fosters a sense of vitality, aliveness, and fulfilment in everyday experiences.

4. Applications of a Somatic mind-set in Everyday Life:

- **Mindful Daily Rituals:** Infuse daily rituals, such as morning routines, meal times, or bedtime rituals, with mindfulness and intention, savoring each moment as an opportunity for presence, connection, and gratitude.

- **Somatic Self-Care:** Prioritize somatic self-care practices, such as relaxation techniques, movement practices, or body awareness exercises, to nurture physical, mental, and emotional well-being and replenish vital energy reserves.

- **Interpersonal Connection:** Apply somatic principles to interpersonal interactions, such as active listening, empathic communication, or non-verbal attunement, fostering deeper connection, understanding, and empathy in relationships.

5. Precautions and Considerations:

- **Gentle Exploration:** Approach the cultivation of a somatic mind-set with gentleness, patience, and self-compassion, recognizing that mindfulness is a skill that develops gradually over time with consistent practice and cultivation.

- **Non-Judgmental Awareness:** Cultivate non-judgmental awareness of thoughts, emotions, and bodily sensations, allowing experiences to unfold with curiosity, acceptance, and kindness, without striving for perfection or control.

- **Integration into Daily Life:** Integrate somatic mind-set practices seamlessly into daily life, finding opportunities for mindfulness and presence in ordinary activities and moments, such as waiting in line, washing dishes, or walking outdoors.

6. Advanced Variations of Cultivating a Somatic mind-set:

- **Embodied Creativity:** Explore embodied creativity as a pathway to self-discovery and expression, engaging in artistic practices, expressive movement, or creative writing as vehicles for somatic exploration and self-expression.

- **Somatic Inquiry:** Cultivate somatic inquiry as a means of deepening self-awareness and insight, investigating habitual patterns, beliefs, and behaviors with curiosity, openness, and self-reflection.

In summary, cultivating a somatic mind-set involves embracing mindfulness, awareness, and presence in every moment of daily life, fostering a deeper connection to oneself, others, and the world around us. By integrating somatic mindset practices into everyday experiences with intention and openness, individuals can enhance overall well-being, authenticity, and fulfillment in their lives.

Chapter 10

Somatic Workout for Long-Term Health and Vitality

Somatic Workout as a Lifelong Practice

Somatic workout is not just a temporary fitness regimen but a lifelong journey towards enhanced health, vitality, and well-being. This section delves into the principles, strategies, benefits, and considerations for integrating somatic workout as a sustainable practice throughout one's life.

1. Understanding Somatic Workout as a Lifelong Practice:

- **Overview:** Somatic workout transcends conventional fitness routines by emphasizing holistic well-being, embodied movement, and mindful awareness as integral components of a lifelong journey towards health and vitality.

- **Purpose:** The primary objective of adopting somatic workout as a lifelong practice is to cultivate sustained physical health, emotional resilience, and mental clarity throughout the lifespan, promoting vitality and well-being at every stage of life.

2. Principles of Lifelong Somatic Practice:

- **Consistency Over Intensity:** Prioritize consistency and sustainability over intensity and duration in somatic workout routines, aiming for regular, manageable practices that can be sustained over the long term.

- **Adaptability and Flexibility:** Embrace adaptability and flexibility in somatic workouts, adjusting practices to accommodate changes in physical abilities, health conditions, or life circumstances as they evolve over time.

- **Mindful Progression:** Progress somatic practices mindfully and gradually, respecting individual limitations and progressing at a pace that feels safe, comfortable, and sustainable for long-term growth and development.

- **Holistic Well-Being:** Approach somatic workout as a holistic practice that integrates physical, mental, emotional, and spiritual dimensions of health and well-being, fostering balance, integration, and harmony in life.

3. Benefits of Lifelong Somatic Practice:

- **Physical Health:** Lifelong somatic practice promotes physical health and vitality by improving flexibility, strength, mobility, and balance, reducing the risk of injury, chronic pain, and age-related decline in physical function.

- **Emotional Resilience:** Somatic practice enhances emotional resilience and well-being by fostering self-awareness, stress management skills, and emotional regulation abilities, enabling individuals to navigate life's challenges with greater ease and equanimity.

- **Mental Clarity:** Regular somatic practice supports mental clarity, focus, and cognitive function by reducing stress, promoting relaxation, and enhancing neural connectivity and plasticity in the brain, fostering cognitive vitality and resilience.

4. Strategies for Sustaining Lifelong Somatic Practice:

- **Mindful Self-Care:** Prioritize self-care practices that support physical, mental, and emotional well-being, such as adequate rest, nourishing nutrition, and stress management techniques, to sustain energy, vitality, and resilience in somatic practice.

- **Community Support:** Engage with a supportive community of like-minded individuals who share a commitment to somatic practice, providing encouragement, accountability, and inspiration for sustaining lifelong growth and development.

- **Professional Guidance:** Seek guidance from qualified somatic practitioners, teachers, or mentors who can offer personalized support, feedback, and guidance to support your journey of lifelong somatic practice with skill and expertise.

- **Lifelong Learning:** Embrace a mindset of lifelong learning and exploration in somatic practice, remaining open to new ideas, perspectives, and approaches that support ongoing growth, discovery, and transformation.

5. Considerations for Lifelong Somatic Practice:

- **Injury Prevention:** Prioritize injury prevention and self-care in somatic practice, listening to your body's signals and respecting its limitations to avoid overexertion, strain, or injury that could impede long-term progress and sustainability.

- **Aging and Adaptation:** Embrace the natural process of aging and adaptation in somatic practice, recognizing that physical abilities, needs, and priorities may change over time and adjusting practices accordingly to support ongoing health and vitality.

- **Self-Compassion:** Cultivate self-compassion and kindness towards yourself in somatic practice, embracing imperfection, setbacks, and challenges as opportunities for growth, learning, and self-discovery along the lifelong journey of health and vitality.

6. Advanced Considerations for Lifelong Somatic Practice:

- **Mind-Body Integration:** Deepen mind-body integration in somatic practice by exploring advanced techniques, such as meditation, visualization, or breathwork, to enhance self-awareness, embodiment, and presence throughout the lifespan.

- **Transpersonal Exploration:** Engage in transpersonal exploration in somatic practice, exploring the interconnectedness of self and cosmos, and cultivating a sense of meaning, purpose, and interconnectedness in life's journey of growth and transformation.

In summary, somatic workout offers a pathway to lifelong health, vitality, and well-being by emphasizing consistency, adaptability, and holistic integration in practice. By embracing somatic practice as a lifelong journey of growth and self-discovery, individuals can cultivate sustained physical health, emotional resilience, and mental clarity, fostering vitality and well-being at every stage of life.

Tracking Progress and Celebrating Achievements

Tracking progress and celebrating achievements are essential components of a long-term somatic workout practice. This section explores the importance of monitoring growth, setting goals, and acknowledging milestones to maintain motivation and sustain progress over time.

1. Understanding the Importance of Tracking Progress:

- **Overview:** Tracking progress involves monitoring changes, improvements, and milestones in somatic practice over time, providing valuable feedback and insights into one's growth and development.

- **Purpose:** The primary objective of tracking progress is to maintain motivation, accountability, and momentum in somatic workout practice by recognizing achievements, identifying areas for growth, and celebrating milestones along the journey.

2. Techniques for Tracking Progress:

- **Goal Setting:** Set specific, measurable, attainable, relevant, and time-bound (SMART) goals for somatic practice, such as increasing flexibility, improving posture, or reducing stress levels, to provide direction and focus for progress tracking.

- **Measurement Tools:** Utilize measurement tools and assessments to track physical, mental, and emotional changes in somatic practice, such as flexibility tests, movement assessments, stress scales, or mood journals, to quantify progress and identify areas for improvement.

- **Progress Journals:** Keep a progress journal or log to record observations, reflections, and insights from somatic practice sessions, noting changes in physical sensations, emotional states, or overall well-being over time.

- **Feedback Loops:** Seek feedback from qualified somatic practitioners, teachers, or mentors to gain external perspective and guidance on progress, receiving constructive feedback, support, and encouragement to enhance growth and development.

3. Benefits of Tracking Progress:

- **Motivation:** Tracking progress fosters motivation and commitment to somatic practice by providing tangible evidence of growth, improvement, and achievement over time, reinforcing positive habits and behaviors.

- **Awareness:** Monitoring progress increases self-awareness and mindfulness in somatic practice, highlighting patterns, trends, and areas for focus and refinement to optimize performance and well-being.

- **Accountability:** Tracking progress holds individuals accountable to their goals and intentions in somatic practice, promoting consistency, discipline, and responsibility in maintaining a regular practice routine.

4. Strategies for Celebrating Achievements:

- **Acknowledge Milestones:** Celebrate achievements and milestones in somatic practice, whether big or small, by acknowledging progress, effort, and dedication with gratitude and appreciation.

- **Reward Yourself:** Reward yourself for reaching goals or milestones in somatic practice, such as treating yourself to a special activity, indulging in self-care, or expressing self-compassion and kindness towards yourself for your accomplishments.

- **Share Successes:** Share successes and achievements with others in your somatic community or support network, celebrating progress and milestones together and inspiring others on their own journey of growth and transformation.

- **Reflect and Integrate:** Reflect on achievements and milestones in somatic practice, integrating lessons learned, insights gained, and successes celebrated into your ongoing journey of growth, learning, and self-discovery.

5. Precautions and Considerations:

- **Avoid Comparison:** Avoid comparing your progress to others in somatic practice, recognizing that each individual's journey is unique and personal, and celebrating your own achievements and milestones with self-compassion and appreciation.

- **Stay Flexible:** Stay flexible and adaptable in goal setting and progress tracking, adjusting expectations and strategies as needed to accommodate changes in circumstances, priorities, or interests over time.

- **Avoid Perfectionism:** Avoid striving for perfectionism in somatic practice, embracing imperfection, setbacks, and challenges as opportunities for growth, learning, and resilience along the journey of long-term health and vitality.

6. Advanced Strategies for Tracking Progress and Celebrating Achievements:

- **Visualization Techniques:** Use visualization techniques to imagine and embody success in somatic practice, visualizing progress, achievements, and goals as if they have already been accomplished, harnessing the power of intention and imagination to manifest desired outcomes.

- **Gratitude Practice:** Cultivate a gratitude practice in somatic workout, expressing gratitude and appreciation for your body, mind, and practice, recognizing the privilege and opportunity of engaging in somatic work for long-term health and vitality.

In summary, tracking progress and celebrating achievements are integral aspects of a long-term somatic workout practice, fostering motivation, accountability, and resilience along the journey of growth and transformation. By setting goals, monitoring progress, and acknowledging milestones with mindfulness and gratitude, individuals can sustain motivation, momentum, and progress in somatic practice, cultivating lifelong health and vitality.

Overcoming Challenges and Setbacks

Somatic workout, like any other practice, comes with its own set of challenges and setbacks. This section delves into strategies for navigating obstacles, overcoming setbacks, and maintaining resilience in pursuit of long-term health and vitality through somatic practice.

1. Understanding Challenges in Somatic Workout:

- **Overview:** Challenges in somatic workout may arise from physical limitations, mental barriers, lack of motivation, or external factors such as time constraints or life stressors.

- **Purpose:** Recognizing and understanding challenges in somatic practice is essential for developing resilience, problem-solving skills, and adaptive strategies to overcome obstacles and setbacks.

2. Common Challenges in Somatic Workout:

- **Physical Discomfort:** Dealing with physical discomfort, pain, or limitations during somatic practice, such as stiffness, tension, or mobility issues, can be a common challenge that requires patience and adaptability to address.

- **Mental Resistance:** Overcoming mental resistance or self-doubt in somatic practice, such as negative thoughts, limiting beliefs, or fear of failure, may hinder progress and require cultivating self-awareness, self-compassion, and positive mindset strategies.

- **Lack of Motivation:** Struggling with lack of motivation or consistency in somatic practice, such as procrastination, boredom, or burnout, may require re-evaluating goals, priorities, and practice routines to reignite passion and commitment.

- **External Obstacles:** Facing external obstacles or barriers to somatic practice, such as time constraints, financial limitations, or environmental factors, may necessitate creative problem-solving, time management skills, and adaptability to navigate challenges effectively.

3. Strategies for Overcoming Challenges:

- **Self-Compassion:** Cultivate self-compassion and kindness towards yourself when facing challenges in somatic practice, acknowledging your efforts, limitations, and humanity with understanding and acceptance.

- **Problem-Solving Skills:** Develop problem-solving skills and resilience in somatic practice, identifying obstacles, generating potential solutions, and implementing action plans to overcome challenges effectively.

- **Support Network:** Seek support from a somatic community, mentor, or coach who can offer guidance, encouragement, and accountability to navigate challenges and setbacks in practice with perspective and wisdom.

- **Adaptive Strategies:** Adopt adaptive strategies and modifications in somatic practice to accommodate limitations, preferences, or changing circumstances, embracing flexibility, creativity, and experimentation in finding solutions that work for you.

4. Benefits of Overcoming Challenges:

- **Personal Growth:** Overcoming challenges in somatic practice fosters personal growth, resilience, and empowerment, building confidence, self-efficacy, and inner strength in facing adversity with courage and determination.

- **Skill Development:** Navigating obstacles and setbacks in somatic practice cultivates valuable skills, such as problem-solving, adaptability, and perseverance, that can be applied to other areas of life for success and fulfillment.

- **Deepened Practice:** Overcoming challenges deepens and enriches somatic practice, offering opportunities for learning, self-discovery, and transformation, and fostering a greater sense of connection, mastery, and fulfillment in the journey of long-term health and vitality.

5. Precautions and Considerations:

- **Avoidance of Pushing Through Pain:** Avoid pushing through pain or discomfort in somatic practice, recognizing the importance of listening to your body's signals and respecting its limitations to prevent injury or exacerbation of symptoms.

- **Balanced Approach:** Maintain a balanced approach to overcoming challenges in somatic practice, acknowledging the importance of persistence, effort, and resilience while also practicing self-care, self-compassion, and self-awareness to ensure sustainable progress and well-being.

- **Seeking Professional Guidance:** Seek guidance from qualified somatic practitioners, teachers, or healthcare providers when facing challenges or setbacks that require specialized knowledge, expertise, or support to address effectively.

6. Advanced Strategies for Overcoming Challenges:

- **Mindfulness and Resilience Training:** Engage in mindfulness and resilience training as complementary practices to somatic workout, cultivating skills in stress management, emotion regulation, and cognitive flexibility to navigate challenges with greater ease and equanimity.

- **Visualization and Affirmations:** Use visualization and affirmations techniques to overcome mental barriers and self-limiting beliefs in somatic practice, imagining success, resilience, and empowerment as if they have already been achieved, harnessing the power of the mind to manifest desired outcomes.

In summary, overcoming challenges and setbacks in somatic workout is an integral part of the journey towards long-term health and vitality. By cultivating resilience, problem-solving skills, and adaptive strategies, individuals can navigate obstacles effectively, deepen their practice, and emerge stronger and more empowered in their pursuit of well-being through somatic practice.

Sharing the Gift of Somatic Movement with Others

Sharing the benefits of somatic movement with others can be a rewarding and enriching experience for both the practitioner and those who receive it. This section explores the various ways in which individuals can share the gift of somatic movement with others to promote health, vitality, and well-being in their communities.

1. Understanding the Power of Sharing Somatic Movement:

- **Overview:** Sharing somatic movement with others involves introducing individuals to the principles and practices of somatic work, empowering them to cultivate greater body awareness, mindfulness, and well-being in their lives.

- **Purpose:** The primary objective of sharing somatic movement is to promote health, vitality, and holistic well-being in individuals and communities, fostering a deeper connection to the body and its innate wisdom and intelligence.

2. Techniques for Sharing Somatic Movement:

- **Teaching and Facilitation:** Become a somatic movement teacher or facilitator, leading classes, workshops, or private sessions to introduce others to somatic principles and practices. Offer guidance, instruction, and support to help individuals explore and embody somatic movement in their own lives.

- **Community Outreach:** Organize community events, outreach programs, or public demonstrations to raise awareness about the benefits of somatic movement and make it accessible to a wider audience. Partner with local organizations, schools, or wellness centers to reach diverse populations and promote inclusivity in somatic practice.

- **Online Platforms:** Utilize online platforms, such as social media, websites, or virtual classes, to share resources, information, and instructional videos on somatic movement. Create online communities or forums where individuals can connect, share experiences, and support each other in their somatic journey.

- **Peer Support:** Offer peer support and mentorship to individuals who are new to somatic movement, providing encouragement, guidance, and accountability to help them integrate somatic practices into their daily lives.

3. Benefits of Sharing Somatic Movement:

- **Empowerment:** Sharing somatic movement empowers individuals to take an active role in their health and well-being, providing them with tools, knowledge, and resources to cultivate greater body awareness, mindfulness, and vitality in their lives.

- **Connection:** Sharing somatic movement fosters a sense of connection and community among individuals, creating opportunities for mutual support, inspiration, and growth in the somatic journey.

- **Transformation:** Sharing somatic movement has the potential to facilitate profound transformation and healing in individuals, addressing physical, mental, and emotional imbalances and promoting holistic well-being and self-discovery.

4. Strategies for Effective Sharing:

- **Cultivate Compassion:** Approach sharing somatic movement with compassion, empathy, and non-judgment, creating a safe and supportive environment where individuals feel valued, respected, and accepted for who they are.

- **Adaptability:** Be adaptable and flexible in your approach to sharing somatic movement, tailoring practices to suit the needs, preferences, and abilities of individuals, and adjusting strategies as needed to accommodate diverse populations and contexts.

- **Communication Skills:** Develop effective communication skills to convey somatic principles and practices clearly and concisely, using language that is accessible, inclusive, and empowering to individuals from all backgrounds and experiences.

- **Lead by Example:** Lead by example in your own somatic practice, embodying the principles of mindfulness, embodiment, and self-care in your daily life, and inspiring others through your commitment, authenticity, and dedication to the somatic journey.

5. Precautions and Considerations:

- **Respect Boundaries:** Respect individuals' boundaries, preferences, and limitations when sharing somatic movement, honoring their autonomy and agency in choosing what feels comfortable and safe for them in their practice.

- **Professional Development:** Continuously invest in professional development and education to enhance your knowledge, skills, and expertise in somatic movement, ensuring that you can offer high-quality, informed guidance and support to those you serve.

- **Ethical Considerations:** Adhere to ethical guidelines and principles in sharing somatic movement, maintaining integrity, transparency, and professionalism in your interactions with others, and prioritizing their well-being and best interests at all times.

6. Advanced Strategies for Sharing Somatic Movement:

- **Community Building:** Foster community building and collaboration among somatic practitioners and enthusiasts, creating opportunities for networking, learning, and growth through shared experiences, events, or initiatives.

- **Research and Advocacy:** Engage in research and advocacy efforts to promote awareness, understanding, and recognition of somatic movement as a valuable and effective approach to health and well-being. Collaborate with researchers, policymakers, and healthcare providers to advocate for greater integration of somatic principles and practices into mainstream healthcare and wellness initiatives.

In summary, sharing the gift of somatic movement with others is a meaningful and impactful way to promote health, vitality, and well-being in individuals and communities. By cultivating compassion, connection, and empowerment, individuals can inspire and support others on their somatic journey, fostering a culture of holistic wellness and self-discovery in society.

Chapter 11

Resources and Further Reading

Recommended Books, Websites, and Online Resources

This chapter provides a curated list of recommended books, websites, and online resources to support continued exploration and learning in somatic movement practices. These resources offer valuable insights, practical guidance, and inspiration for integrating somatic principles into daily life and promoting long-term health and vitality.

1. Recommended Books:

- **"Somatics: Reawakening The Mind's Control Of Movement, Flexibility, And Health" by Thomas Hanna:** This seminal book offers a comprehensive introduction to somatic movement principles, exploring the mind-body connection and providing practical exercises for improving movement, flexibility, and overall well-being.

- **"The Mindful Body: Build Emotional Strength and Manage Stress with Body Mindfulness" by Noa Belling:** This book combines mindfulness practices with somatic movement techniques to promote emotional resilience, stress management, and self-awareness through embodied mindfulness.

- **"Dynamic Alignment Through Imagery" by Eric Franklin:** This book introduces imagery-based techniques for enhancing movement quality, alignment, and proprioception, integrating somatic principles with visualization exercises to improve performance and prevent injury.

- **"The Thinking Body: A Study of the Balancing Forces of Dynamic Man" by Mabel Elsworth Todd:** Originally published in 1937, this classic text explores the principles of dynamic balance and coordination, offering insights into the relationship between movement, perception, and consciousness.

2. Websites and Online Resources:

- **Somatics.org:** This website offers a wealth of information on somatic practices, including articles, videos, and resources for exploring somatic movement, therapy, and education.

- **SomaticMovementCenter.com:** Founded by Martha Peterson, a certified clinical somatic educator, this website provides online courses, workshops, and resources for learning clinical somatic education techniques to relieve chronic pain, improve posture, and enhance movement efficiency.

- **The Mindful Body:** This website offers a range of resources for integrating mindfulness and somatic practices into daily life, including guided meditations, yoga classes, and articles on mindfulness-based stress reduction and somatic experiencing.

- **SomaticsToolkit.com:** This website features a collection of somatic exercises, movement sequences, and educational resources for self-care, relaxation, and embodied awareness, curated by somatic movement educators and practitioners.

3. Online Courses and Workshops:

- **Mindful Somatics Institute:** This online institute offers courses and workshops in mindfulness-based somatic practices, including embodied mindfulness, somatic yoga, and movement meditation for cultivating presence and well-being.

- **Somatic Systems Institute:** Founded by Thomas Hanna, the Somatic Systems Institute offers online training programs in clinical somatic education, providing certification courses for individuals interested in becoming somatic educators and practitioners.

- **The Feldenkrais Method®:** Developed by Moshe Feldenkrais, the Feldenkrais Method® offers online classes, workshops, and training programs in somatic movement education, focusing on improving movement quality, flexibility, and awareness through gentle, exploratory movement sequences.

- **Dynamic Embodiment™:** Created by Dr. Martha Eddy, Dynamic Embodiment™ offers online courses and workshops in somatic movement therapy and education, integrating principles from somatic psychology, dance/movement therapy, and body-mind centering.

4. Social Media Communities:

- **Instagram:** Follow somatic movement practitioners, educators, and organizations on Instagram for daily inspiration, tips, and resources for integrating somatic practices into your life.

- **Facebook Groups:** Join somatic movement and mindfulness communities on Facebook to connect with like-minded individuals, share experiences, and participate in discussions on somatic practices, techniques, and resources.

- **YouTube Channels:** Subscribe to YouTube channels dedicated to somatic movement, yoga, meditation, and mindfulness for instructional videos, guided practices, and demonstrations of somatic exercises and techniques.

In conclusion, these recommended books, websites, online resources, courses, and social media communities offer valuable support and guidance for deepening your understanding and practice of somatic movement. Whether you are new to somatics or an experienced practitioner, these resources provide opportunities for continued exploration, learning, and growth in promoting long-term health and vitality through somatic practices.

Finding Somatic Movement Classes and Workshops

In this section, we explore various avenues for finding somatic movement classes and workshops, both in-person and online. These resources provide opportunities for hands-on learning, guided practice, and community support in exploring somatic principles and techniques for enhancing health and well-being.

1. Local Studios and Wellness Centers:

- **Search Online Directories:** Use online directories such as Google Maps, Yelp, or Mindbody to search for local studios, wellness centers, or gyms that offer somatic movement classes and workshops in your area.

- **Contact Studios Directly:** Reach out to local studios and wellness centers to inquire about their class offerings, schedules, and instructors. Ask about introductory classes, trial sessions, or special events to experience somatic movement firsthand.

2. Yoga and Pilates Studios:

- **Check Class Schedules:** Many yoga and Pilates studios offer somatic movement classes as part of their regular class schedules. Look for classes labeled as "somatic yoga," "somatic movement," or "somatics" to explore somatic principles within the context of these practices.

- **Attend Workshops and Events:** Yoga and Pilates studios often host workshops, retreats, and special events focused on somatic movement. Keep an eye on their event calendars or sign up for their newsletters to stay informed about upcoming opportunities.

3. Community Centers and Recreation Programs:

- **Explore Community Offerings:** Community centers, recreation programs, and adult education centers sometimes offer somatic movement classes as part of their health and wellness programming. Check their class catalogs or websites for information on upcoming sessions.

- **Attend Free or Low-Cost Events:** Look for free or low-cost events, such as wellness fairs, health expos, or community outreach programs, where somatic movement instructors may offer introductory workshops or demonstrations.

4. Online Platforms and Streaming Services:

- **Subscription Services:** Explore subscription-based platforms such as Yoga International, Gaia, or

Mindvalley for online somatic movement classes, workshops, and courses led by experienced instructors from around the world.

- **Social Media Platforms:** Follow somatic movement practitioners and instructors on social media platforms such as Instagram, Facebook, or YouTube for access to free or paid online classes, tutorials, and live streams.

5. Specialized Somatic Movement Schools and Institutes:

- **Somatic Education Programs:** Consider enrolling in somatic education programs offered by specialized schools and institutes, such as the Somatic Systems Institute, the Mindful Somatics Institute, or the Feldenkrais Method® Training Programs.

- **Certification Courses:** If you are interested in becoming a certified somatic movement instructor or practitioner, explore certification courses and training programs offered by accredited organizations and professional associations in the field of somatics.

6. Online Directories and Class Listings:

- **Somatic Movement Directories:** Search online directories and class listings specifically dedicated to somatic movement practices, such as Somatics.org or the International Somatic Movement Education and Therapy Association (ISMETA) website, for information on classes, workshops, and events worldwide.

- **Event Platforms:** Check event platforms such as Eventbrite or Meetup for listings of somatic movement classes, workshops, and gatherings in your area or online.

In summary, finding somatic movement classes and workshops is accessible through various avenues, including local studios, wellness centers, online platforms, specialized schools, and community resources. Whether you prefer in-person instruction or online learning, there are abundant opportunities to explore somatic principles and techniques for promoting health, vitality, and well-being in your daily life.

Somatic Workout Communities and Support Groups

This section delves into the importance of somatic workout communities and support groups and offers guidance on how to find and engage with them. These communities provide valuable opportunities for connection, encouragement, and shared learning in the journey towards improved health and well-being through somatic practices.

1. Importance of Somatic Workout Communities:

- **Sense of Belonging:** Somatic workout communities foster a sense of belonging and connection among individuals who share an interest in somatic practices, creating a supportive environment where members can learn, grow, and thrive together.

- **Encouragement and Accountability:** Being part of a somatic workout community provides opportunities for mutual encouragement and accountability, motivating members to stay committed to their practice and goals through shared experiences and support.

- **Learning and Sharing:** Communities offer platforms for learning and sharing knowledge, insights, and resources related to somatic movement practices, enriching members' understanding and practice through diverse perspectives and experiences.

2. Finding Somatic Workout Communities:

- **Local Meetup Groups:** Search for local meetup groups or gatherings focused on somatic movement, mindfulness, or holistic health in your area. Joining these groups allows you to connect with like-minded individuals and participate in community events, workshops, or practice sessions.

- **Online Forums and Social Media:** Explore online forums, social media groups, and discussion boards dedicated to somatic workout practices. Platforms like Facebook, Reddit, or specialized forums provide opportunities to engage with a global community of practitioners, share resources, and seek advice or support.

- **Somatic Movement Organizations:** Look for professional organizations or associations dedicated to somatic movement education and therapy, such as ISMETA (International Somatic Movement Education and Therapy Association). These organizations often offer membership benefits, networking opportunities, and community events for practitioners and enthusiasts.

- **Studio or Class Communities:** Engage with the community of practitioners at local studios, wellness centers, or gyms that offer somatic workout classes. Attend classes regularly, participate in studio events or workshops, and connect with fellow participants to build relationships and support networks within the studio community.

3. Engaging with Somatic Workout Communities:

- **Active Participation:** Actively participate in somatic workout communities by attending events, joining discussions, and sharing your experiences and insights with fellow members. Contribute to the community by offering support, guidance, or resources to others.

- **Seeking Mentorship:** Seek out mentors or experienced practitioners within the community who can provide guidance, encouragement, and mentorship in your somatic practice journey. Build relationships with mentors through formal mentorship programs, informal mentoring arrangements, or one-on-one coaching sessions.

- **Organizing Community Events:** Take initiative in organizing community events, workshops, or gatherings focused on somatic workout practices. Collaborate with fellow practitioners or community leaders to create opportunities for shared learning, practice, and connection within the community.

- **Online Engagement:** Stay engaged with online somatic workout communities through regular participation in discussions, sharing of resources, and collaboration on projects or initiatives. Contribute positively to the community culture by fostering inclusivity, respect, and support among members.

4. Benefits of Somatic Workout Communities:

- **Support and Encouragement:** Somatic workout communities offer a supportive environment where members can receive encouragement, feedback, and validation from peers, fostering motivation and resilience in their practice.

- **Shared Learning:** Communities provide opportunities for shared learning and exploration of somatic practices, allowing members to benefit from diverse perspectives, experiences, and insights within the community.

- **Connection and Friendship:** Being part of a somatic workout community fosters connections and friendships with like-minded individuals who share common interests and values, enriching members' social and emotional well-being.

- **Collaboration and Growth:** Communities inspire collaboration and growth through collective learning, innovation, and creativity, empowering members to expand their horizons, challenge themselves, and reach new levels of proficiency and mastery in somatic practice.

In summary, somatic workout communities and support groups play a crucial role in fostering connection, encouragement, and shared learning among practitioners. By actively engaging with these communities, individuals can enhance their somatic practice experience, build meaningful relationships, and cultivate a sense of belonging and empowerment in their journey towards improved health and vitality through somatic movement.

Continuing Education and Professional Development Opportunities

This section explores the various avenues for continuing education and professional development in the field of somatic movement. Whether you're a novice practitioner seeking to deepen your understanding or an experienced professional looking to expand your skill set, these opportunities offer valuable resources for growth and advancement in somatic practices.

1. Advanced Training Programs:

- **Somatic Movement Education:** Enroll in advanced training programs in somatic movement education offered by accredited institutions or professional organizations. These programs provide in-depth study of somatic principles, advanced techniques, and specialized applications in areas such as clinical somatic education, dance/movement therapy, or somatic psychology.

- **Certification Courses:** Pursue certification courses in specific somatic modalities or approaches, such as the Feldenkrais Method®, Alexander Technique, or Body-Mind Centering®. These certification programs typically involve comprehensive training, supervised practice, and assessment to ensure proficiency and competency in the respective modality.

2. Workshops and Intensive Retreats:

- **Specialized Workshops:** Attend workshops and intensive retreats led by renowned somatic practitioners, educators, and experts. These short-term programs offer focused exploration of specific topics, techniques, or applications within somatic movement, providing opportunities for immersive learning and skill development.

- **Continuing Education Credits:** Look for workshops and retreats that offer continuing education credits or professional development units for somatic movement practitioners, therapists, or educators. These credits may be required for maintaining certification or licensure in certain professions.

3. Online Courses and Webinars:

- **E-Learning Platforms:** Explore online courses, webinars, and virtual workshops offered by reputable institutions, organizations, or individual practitioners in somatic movement. These online learning platforms provide flexible and accessible opportunities for self-paced study, interactive learning, and skill acquisition in somatic practices.

- **Specialized Topics:** Seek out online courses and webinars that cover specialized topics or emerging trends in somatic movement, such as trauma-informed somatics, embodied mindfulness, or somatic experiencing. These courses offer insights and strategies for addressing specific client populations or therapeutic issues within somatic practice.

4. Mentorship and Supervision:

- **Mentorship Programs:** Participate in mentorship programs or apprenticeships with experienced somatic practitioners, educators, or therapists. Mentorship offers personalized guidance, feedback, and support in developing clinical skills, professional competencies, and ethical practice in somatic movement.

- **Supervision and Consultation:** Seek supervision or consultation from seasoned professionals in the field of somatic movement therapy or education. Supervision provides opportunities for reflective practice, case consultation, and professional development, enhancing clinical competence and effectiveness in working with clients.

5. Conferences and Symposiums:

- **Professional Conferences:** Attend national or international conferences dedicated to somatic movement, mindfulness, or body-oriented therapies. These conferences feature keynote presentations, workshops, research presentations, and networking opportunities for connecting with peers, staying informed about current trends, and expanding professional networks.

- **Interdisciplinary Exchange:** Explore interdisciplinary conferences or symposiums that bring together professionals from diverse fields such as psychology, neuroscience, dance/movement therapy, and bodywork. These events provide opportunities for cross-disciplinary dialogue, collaboration, and innovation in somatic practices.

6. Research and Publication:

- **Literature Review:** Stay updated on the latest research and literature in somatic movement by regularly reviewing academic journals, books, and publications in the field. Subscribe to relevant journals or online databases for access to scholarly articles, research studies, and theoretical frameworks in somatics.

- **Contributions to the Field:** Consider contributing to the field of somatic movement through research, writing, or publication. Share your insights, experiences, and findings through academic papers, journal articles, book chapters, or online blogs to contribute to the ongoing dialogue and advancement of somatic practices.

In summary, continuing education and professional development opportunities in somatic movement offer diverse avenues for growth, learning, and advancement in the field. By actively engaging with these opportunities, practitioners can deepen their knowledge, refine their skills, and stay connected with the evolving landscape of somatic practices, ultimately enhancing their effectiveness and impact as somatic movement professionals.

www.ingramcontent.com/pod-product-compliance
Lightning Source LLC
Chambersburg PA
CBHW070831250726
48662CB00003B/1171